Nutritarian Handbook
& FOOD SCORING GUIDE

Heal your body and transform your life at Dr. Fuhrman's

EAT TO LIVE RETREAT

San Diego County, California

At the Eat to Live Retreat, Dr. Fuhrman and his expert team will help you take control of your health. Drawing on his 30+ years of experience practicing lifestyle medicine, Dr. Fuhrman will design a plan that will help you lose excess weight, reverse chronic disease, reduce / eliminate medications, and end addictive food behaviors.

This immersive experience includes delicious and organic Nutritarian meals prepared by expert chefs, cooking classes with our chefs, lectures by Dr. Fuhrman, group fitness classes that are individualized based on a person's strength and balance, group sessions to discuss emotional eating and food addition, water aerobics in our heated salt-water pool, yoga, our relaxing jacuzzi, games galore and more. Our entire staff, including our house manager and full-time nurse, make sure your stay is a life-changing experience. You will go home with the knowledge and strategies to continue your journey to a healthy, long and vibrant life.

Find out more about this beautiful residential facility, located just 30 minutes north of downtown San Diego, by visiting DrFuhrman.com/etlretreat or call (949) 432-6295.

Nutritarian Handbook
& FOOD SCORING GUIDE

JOEL FUHRMAN, M.D.

PUBLISHED BY

ɕɧɒ

Gift of Health Press

First Edition, Published by Gift of Health Press, 2012

Second Edition
COPYRIGHT 2012, 2022 BY JOEL FUHRMAN, M.D
All Rights Reserved

Contact:
Gift of Health Press
Flemington, NJ 08822
for wholesale inquiries go to:
giftofhealthpress.com

Printed in the United States of America
ISBN: 978-1-7356072-8-3
Library of Congress Control Number: 2022911463

Publisher's Note:
Do not start, stop, or change medication without professional medical advice, and do not change your diet if you are ill or on medication, except under the supervision of a competent physician. Neither this, nor any other book, is intended to take the place of personalized medical care or treatment.

ꝗꝒ
Gift of Health Press

CONTENTS

INTRODUCTION

No one wants to have a heart attack, suffer a debilitating stroke or develop cancer. But lots of people die from these conditions every day... unnecessarily.

Nutritional science has made dramatic advances in recent years. The overwhelming accumulation of scientific knowledge points to a dramatic conclusion—the majority of diseases plaguing Americans are preventable. Using the information compiled from scientific studies, it is now possible to formulate a few simple diet and lifestyle principles that can save you years of suffering and premature death. You have an unprecedented opportunity in human history to enjoy better health and live longer than ever before.

But being in the best of health and living longer comes at a price.

How much would it be worth to you for a guarantee that you would never have a heart attack or a stroke? What would it be worth to you to healthfully and happily watch your children and grandchildren grow? What would you be willing to pay for the assurance that you would not leave your spouse or your children all alone?

Fortunately, the expenditure is infinitely affordable—little more than the effort needed to establish new, more healthful eating habits.

Everything in this book is supported by the preponderance of evidence from scientific studies. Still, the facts and guidelines will astound most physicians. Although the research is readily available for all to see, most people still have no idea that food can be the most powerful weapon in the fight against the major illnesses that plague our society. Now is the time for you to open your eyes to the value of superior nutrition, put wholesome food in your body and take control of your health destiny.

1

AMERICA'S HEALTH CRISIS AND YOU

Americans are digging their graves with their knives and forks. It is not news that Americans are sickly and fat; almost everybody knows that modern America is in the midst of an all-you-can eat food fest that has us literally bursting at the seams. We are not only eating ourselves into sickness and premature death – we also have a health care crisis with upward-spiraling medical care costs. The economic costs of heart disease and other diet-related chronic diseases are staggering.

The National Health Expenditure Accounts (NHEA) are the official estimates of total health care spending in the United States. In 1960, health care spending in the United States totaled $27.2 billion. By 2000, total health expenditures had reached about $1.4 trillion; in 2018, the amount spent had more than doubled to $3.6 trillion.[1] In

2020, health care spending in the United States rose to $4.1 trillion or $12,530 per person. As a share of the nation's Gross Domestic Product, health spending accounted for 19.7 percent.[2]

Excess fat is detrimental at any level. Health care costs increase in parallel with body mass index (BMI), even beginning in the range of recommended BMIs.[3] These out-of-control costs play an important role in business failures, bankruptcies and loss of jobs. Our health system relies on an ever-expanding arsenal of medications, tests and procedures that fail to address the root cause of our escalating ill health: the way we choose to eat and live. In America, we have attempted to solve our diet-caused health woes with the development of multiple medications for diabetes, hypertension and cholesterol-lowering. We have heart procedures and surgeries, all at a dramatic expense. We have been led to believe that drugs and doctors save lives, but the statistics show otherwise – lifespan is not significantly enhanced by the vast majority of medical interventions.

The Obesity Epidemic

Diseases caused by nutrition are now the largest causes of death throughout the world.[4] For the first time globally, the number of overweight individuals rivals the number of those who are underweight. In recent years, the growth of processed foods, convenience foods and fast foods has supplied our relatively sedentary society with a diet of high-calorie foods that contain few nutrients. In all parts of the world, obesity appears to escalate as income increases and fast food and processed foods become available. In the United States, being overweight is the norm, and almost all adults eventually take medications for diabetes, cholesterol and/or blood pressure. By 2018, the prevalence of obesity in the U.S. was 42.4%, increasing from 30.5% in 2000. At the same time, the rate of severe obesity (BMI of 40 or greater) rose from 4.7% to 9.2%.[5]

Obesity is a major risk factor associated with highly prevalent and serious diseases such as heart disease, cancer and diabetes. The diet-style that creates these diseases fuels out-of-control medical costs. Seventy-eight percent of Americans today are overweight or obese, up from 46 percent in 1960.[6] The average American today weighs almost 30 pounds more than they did in the 1960s,[7, 8] and has a considerably higher risk of heart attack, stroke and cancer to show for it.

Health Complications of Obesity

- Increased overall mortality
- Type 2 diabetes
- Hypertension
- Degenerative arthritis
- Coronary artery disease
- Obstructive sleep apnea
- Gallstones
- Fatty infiltration of liver
- Restrictive lung disease
- Cancer

Poor Nutrition Everywhere

In the 20th century, processed foods became increasingly prevalent in the average American diet. The consumption of fresh produce and whole grains plummeted, while the consumption of animal products increased. As a result, Americans now consume far more calories, fat, cholesterol, refined sugar, animal protein, sodium, and white flour, and far less whole plant foods, with all their fiber and plant-derived nutrients, than is healthful. As a result, obesity, diabetes, heart disease and cancer have skyrocketed.

CHANGES IN FOOD CONSUMPTION IN THE UNITED STATES, 1900-2020[9-12]

	1900	2020
Sugar	5 lbs/year	72.7 lbs/year
Soft drinks	0	38.9 gallons/year
Oils	4 lbs/year	51.7 lbs/year
Cheese	2 lbs/year	28.2 lbs/year
Meat	140 lbs/year	148.1 lbs/year
Calories	2100/day	2500-3800/day

The meat and poultry industries are the largest segment of U.S. agriculture. Meat production in the U.S. totaled 52 billion pounds in 2017, and U.S. poultry production totaled 48 billion pounds in 2017.[13]

It is clear that the average American is eating themselves to death. A diet centered on meat, cheese, and sugar-filled snacks, within the groundwork of calorie overload, lays the foundation for obesity, cancer, heart disease, diabetes, and autoimmune illnesses.

It is not solely that these foods are harmful; it is also what we are not eating that is causing the problem. We are not eating enough nutrient-rich produce. When you calculate all the calories consumed from the standard American diet, you find that the calories coming from the most health-promoting foods, such as fresh fruit, vegetables (not including white potatoes), beans, raw nuts, and seeds, represent only about 13% of the total caloric intake. This dangerously low intake of unrefined plant foods is what guarantees weakened immunity to infectious disease, frequent illnesses and a shorter lifespan. We will never win the war on cancer, heart disease, diabetes, and other degenerative illnesses unless we address this deficiency. Though the American diet has spread all over the world, bringing with it heart disease, cancer and obesity, studies still show that in the populations that eat more fruits and vegetables, the incidences of death from these diseases is dramatically lowered.

COMPOSITION OF THE AMERICAN DIET

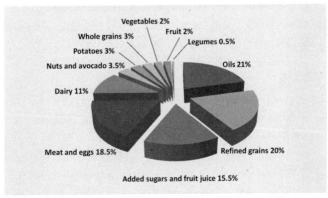

Vegetables 2%
Fruit 2%
Whole grains 3%
Legumes 0.5%
Potatoes 3%
Nuts and avocado 3.5%
Oils 21%
Dairy 11%
Meat and eggs 18.5%
Refined grains 20%
Added sugars and fruit juice 15.5%

United States Department of Agriculture. Economic Research Service. Food Availability (Per Capita) Data System https://www.ers.usda.gov/data-products/food-availability-per-capita-data-system/food-availability-per-capita-data-system/

Heart Disease is Preventable

Heart disease is a much bigger problem than most people think. It is the leading cause of death for both men and women in the U.S. It affects almost all Americans, with one in four adults over the age of 40, and more than 40% of adults over the age of 60, taking prescription cholesterol-lowering medication.[14] Yet heart disease is one of the top preventable causes of death. Modern medical techniques and drugs cannot win this war, because the true cause of disease is overlooked. Heart disease, and most other common modern diseases, are caused by inadequate nutrition. The tragedy is enormous. And when you consider that nobody really has to die from a heart- or circulatory system-related death, it is even more of a tragedy. The disability, suffering and years of life lost are almost totally the result of dietary ignorance. It is not impossible or even difficult to protect yourself; you simply must eat properly. Nothing else can offer such dramatic protection.

4 Simple Truths

While America's health crisis is real, you can reclaim your health. Consider these four critical points:

- We are brainwashed into thinking that drugs are the answer to our health problems

- Unhealthy food is addictive

- Foods that don't contain health-promoting micronutrients lead to overeating

- A normal body weight in conjunction with nutritional adequacy is essential for good health and longevity

Understanding these simple truths is the key to solving the health care problems of most Americans. The cells in our bodies need a wide array of nutrients, numbering in the thousands, to function normally. The human body is designed to be fueled by natural, nutrient-rich plant food. Foods supply not just vitamins and minerals, but also thousands of immune-supporting substances

9

called phytochemicals that are essential for our protection against disease. While science has described these needs, an astonishing percentage of Americans do not meet the recommended intakes for vitamins and minerals. For example, only about 45 percent of Americans meet the recommended intake for magnesium, 60 percent meet it for for vitamin E, and 35 percent meet it for for vitamin K.[15, 16] Very few people eat healthfully enough to protect themselves against disease in later life.

Why Diets Fail

Low-nutrient eating drives overeating behavior, and is the primary cause of obesity, disease and death in the modern world. Have you ever been on a diet, losing and gaining the same 10, 20 or 30 pounds? The number of people who successfully lose weight through dieting and keep it off for the rest of their lives is fewer than one out of five. The other 80-85% of people who lose weight gain it back, which is often unhealthier than not losing it at all.[17, 18]

The biggest problem with most diets is that you are asked to deprive yourself using portion control, low carbs, fewer calories, etc. Deprivation never works, and your food cravings return with a vengeance! This is the basis of the "yo-yo" dieting industry. I want you to know that it's not that you have failed a diet; it's that the system (diets, magic pills, surgeries, etc.) has failed you. My findings, based on more than three decades of experience with over 10,000 patients, and thousands of supportive research studies, is that a properly nourished body will seek its ideal weight. So instead of "dieting," I want to show you the foods that provide the nutrition your body needs. The body has an incredible ability to heal itself and get back in balance when you feed it what it needs. It's that simple! Your body is like a supercomputer: Feed it right, and it will keep you fit, lean and healthy.

Enjoy a Full, More Pleasurable Life

If you are reading this, it is likely that you are someone who is ready to take control of your health. Superior nutrition is the foundation of this diet. It is the path to medical wellness in your life. It is the most powerful intervention, not only to prevent disease, but to also reverse it. Complete recovery from most chronic degenerative illnesses is possible.

The information presented here is the fastest and most effective way to create an optimal nutritional environment for self-healing. This plant-based, high-nutrient diet can enable you to avoid angioplasty, bypass surgery and other invasive procedures. By adopting this eating style, you can protect yourself against heart attack, stroke and dementia. You can reduce and eventually eliminate your need for prescription drugs. You will not only optimize your health and potentially save your life; this eating style will also increase the pleasure you get from food. It will result in the lessening of hunger, the removal of addiction, and – if needed – profound and long-term weight loss. I have seen this in my medical practice and it has been documented in a medical publication.[19] Millions of people have read Eat to Live and have learned how to take control of their health destiny. At our Eat to Live Retreat, my wife Lisa and I witness marvelous health transformations; in some cases, even we are amazed. As Lisa has said many times over, our guests "turn back the clock" physically and mentally.

When you supply your body with optimal nutrition, it knows how to heal itself. That is the main premise of all my work. Your body has tremendous healing powers when given the right foods. Unleashing your body's power to work optimally brings energy back into your life. You will not only reach your ideal body weight, but you will enjoy a longer, more healthful and more pleasurable life.

More and more, new medical studies are investigating and demonstrating that diets rich in high-nutrient plant foods have a suppressive effect on appetite and are most effective for long-term weight control.[20-24] The healthiest way to eat is also the most successful way to obtain a favorable weight, if you consider long-term results. I am thrilled to be able to work with you and address your diet-related health issues. You will learn how to feed your body so that it operates at its highest level every day. Your energy levels will soar to new heights, without relying on artificial stimulants like coffee and sugar. You will sleep better; your skin will look better, and you will feel and look younger. In short, your properly nourished body will allow you to live life to the fullest!

I encourage you to read any or all my books - Eat to Live, Disease-Proof Your Child, Eat for Health, The End of Dieting, The End of Heart Disease, The End of Diabetes, Super Immunity, Fast Food Genocide, and my latest book, Eat for Life - for a more comprehensive understanding and application of these principles. A good place to start is my most recent work: Eat for Life. I also offer an assortment of valuable membership features at www.DrFuhrman.com, where you can obtain more detailed, personalized nutritional guidance and support.

2

BECOMING A NUTRITARIAN

Not Your Typical Diet

Typical diet books usually contain a list of rules and regulations to restrict calories for weight loss. This is a problem, because when the focus is weight loss alone, results are rarely permanent. The focus in this handbook is on nutrition and eating healthfully, which is an undisputed, yet often overlooked critical ingredient for any dietary success. Here, there is no carbohydrate, protein, fat or calorie counting or weighing involved. In fact, you will eat as much food as you want and still, over time, become healthier and satisfied with fewer calories. Your properly nourished body will automatically seek its ideal weight, without having to fight the scale or count calories.

The fundamentals of this eating style are to increase high-nutrient foods in your diet and to "crowd out" unhealthful, low-nutrient foods. What does it mean to "crowd out"? It means that as you eat more delicious, high-nutrient foods, you will be reducing your desire for fatty, processed and unhealthful products.

When you change the foods you eat to better meet your nutrient needs, you feel better and it eventually becomes your preferred way of eating. To accomplish this, you will be presented with scientific, logical information that explains the connection between food, your weight and your health.

If you need to lose weight, this information will help you shed pounds naturally and easily, merely as a side effect of eating so healthfully.

What is a Nutritarian?

When you learn and practice this eating style, you can proudly call yourself a Nutritarian. A Nutritarian is someone who strives to consume, and learns to prefer foods that are nutritious. Quite simply, a Nutritarian:

- Eats mainly high-nutrient, natural plant foods: vegetables, fruits, beans, nuts and seeds.

- Eats few, if any, animal products (one or two servings per week at most) and chooses healthier options in this food group.

- Avoids foods that are completely empty of nutrients or toxic for the body, such as sugar, sweeteners, white flour, processed foods and fast foods.

The Nutritarian way to health, longevity and weight loss focuses on the healthy foods with the strongest evidence supporting their anti-cancer and longevity-promoting effects. Remember this acronym:

G-BOMBS
*Greens, Beans, Onions, Mushrooms, Berries and Seeds
=> Foods that promote DNA repair and healing*

Green vegetables, particularly leafy green cruciferous vegetables, along with beans, onions, mushrooms, berries, and seeds, are the foods that have documented benefits to prevent cancer and other diseases. Of course, all micronutrient-rich foods help prevent these illnesses, but these foods have the strongest scientific evidence demonstrating protection against cancer, and should be eaten daily.

A Nutritarian is someone who learns to trust the amazing power of the body. If given the chance, the body will heal itself, with the right food as the catalyst.

When you become a Nutritarian, you will arm yourself with the biochemical sustenance that your body needs to be at its ideal weight and to live a healthy, empowered life.

Finally, a Nutritarian lifestyle is an attitude, a mindset, a method that can be followed for a lifetime. As you begin your journey as a Nutritarian, you will be empowered to take control of your own health and life.

Vegan, Vegetarian, Nutritarian

The foundation of the Nutritarian diet is vegetables and other high-nutrient foods, but it does not have to be at the exclusion of all animal foods. A vegan diet is one that contains no foods of animal product origin, whereas a vegetarian diet may contain some dairy and eggs. A vegetarian or vegan diet can be an option for excellent health, as long as care is taken to eat healthful, nutrient-rich foods.

However, a vegetarian or vegan who lives on processed cereals, white flour products, white rice, white potato and processed soy products is still vulnerable to the weight gain and diseases resulting from the standard American diet, because their diet cannot be considered nutrient-rich.

Being a Nutritarian differs from being a typical vegan because the focus isn't on totally excluding animal foods. The focus is on including the high-nutrient foods a body needs to improve health dramatically. A Nutritarian can reduce the intake of animal products to a safe level without having to exclude them completely. A Nutritarian could be a vegan or not. Eating this way makes either option healthful.

The Nutritarian Difference

The Nutritarian diet is different because it doesn't require deprivation, starvation or denying your body foods that properly nourish it. It truly is a whole new way of looking at food. This handbook will show you why nutrient-rich foods are so powerful, and will help you learn exactly what to eat and how to incorporate these foods into your diet.

Your body can change in amazing and dramatic ways. Thousands, if not millions of people who have adopted the Nutritarian lifestyle have reversed diet-related diseases such as diabetes, heart disease, chronic fatigue, autoimmune disease and migraines.

The right food can be the most healing "medicine" you put in your body. Whether you want to lose weight or just eat more healthfully, an easy way to make the right dietary choices is to sort foods into three categories:

Eat Liberally

Eat in Moderation

Avoid Entirely

Note that the term "eat liberally" is more accurate than the term "unlimited." Unlimited could imply overeating, or recreational or emotional eating, or eating when not hungry. Also, consuming too much of a very healthy food, such as fruit, can lead to insufficient vegetables in your diet.

The Nutritarian diet encourages liberal consumption of raw vegetables, cooked green and non-green, nutrient-dense vegetables, fruit, and beans. Raw nuts and seeds are included in the diet, but in limited quantities if weight loss is a goal. Starchy vegetables and whole grains are also included in the diet, but in limited amounts.

Products made with refined sugar and refined white flour are off-limits, as well as barbecued, processed and cured meat, and all red meat and cheese. These foods are deficient in micronutrients, and do not contain antioxidants and phytochemicals, thus decreasing the nutrient density of your diet. Significant quantities of high-protein animal products also drive up hormones linked to higher rates of breast, prostate and colon cancer.

Foods to Eat Liberally, Eat in Moderation, or Avoid Entirely

Eat Liberally

You can eat as much as you want of these foods (within reason):

- **Raw vegetables** *(Goal: about 1 pound daily)*
- **Cooked green and non-green, nutrient-dense vegetables** *(Goal: about ½ to 1 pound daily)* Non-green, nutrient-dense veggies are: tomatoes, cauliflower, eggplant, mushrooms, peppers, onions and carrots
- **Beans, legumes, lentils, tempeh, edamame, tofu** *(Goal: 1/2 to 1 cup daily)*
- **Fresh or frozen fruit** *(3 to 5 servings per day; 1 serving should be berries. One serving = 1 piece or 1 to 1 ½ cups berries or chopped fruit.)*

Limited (Eat in Moderation)

Include these foods in your diet but limit the amount you are eating.

- **Cooked starchy vegetables or whole grains** *(Maximum: 2 servings daily; 1 serving = 1 cup or 1 slice; limit bread items to no more than 3 servings per week)*
  - Butternut and other winter squashes
  - Potatoes, corn or wild rice
  - Quinoa other intact whole grains
  - 100% whole grain bread
- **Raw nuts and seeds** Half should be walnuts or chia, hemp, flax or sesame seeds *(Eat at least 1 ounce or ¼ cup per day; if trying to lose weight, limit to a maximum of 1.5 ounces for women and 2 ounces for men per day)*
- **Avocado** *(Maximum ½ per day)*
- **Dried Fruit** *(Maximum 2 tablespoons per day)*
- **Animal Products** unsweetened fat-free dairy (skim milk, fat-free yogurt), wild fish and certified organic poultry *(Maximum of 6 ounces per week, limit each serving size to 2 ounces and use as a minor component/flavoring agent).*

Note: *If you are not trying to lose weight, amounts of cooked starchy vegetables, intact whole grains, nuts, seeds and avocado may be increased depending on your caloric needs.*

Off-Limits

- **Products made with white sugar, white flour, honey, or maple syrup**
- **Soda and soft drinks** including those made with artificial sweeteners
- **Fruit Juice** (except pomegranate juice)
- **Barbecued, processed and cured meats and all red meat**
- **Full-fat and reduced-fat dairy** (cheese, ice cream, butter, milk)
- **Egg yolks**
- **Oils such as olive oil and other vegetable oil**

Note: *If you are not trying to lose weight, a small amount of olive oil may be used – but aim for a maximum of 1 tablespoon/week. See recommendations on Page 48.*

CHAPTER THREE

THE HEALTH EQUATION

Discovering Nutrients

There are two kinds of nutrients: macronutrients and micronutrients. The calorie-containing macronutrients are protein, carbohydrate, and fat. Water is also a macronutrient, but contains no calories.

Micronutrients are vitamins, minerals and phytochemicals, and are calorie-free. Obviously, we need to consume both kinds of nutrients, but the American diet contains too many macronutrients and not enough micronutrients.

MACRONUTRIENTS = FAT, CARBOHYDRATES & PROTEIN
(CONTAIN CALORIES)
SHOULD LIMIT CONSUMPTION

MICRONUTRIENTS = VITAMINS, MINERALS & PHYTOCHEMICALS
DO NOT CONTAIN CALORIES
SHOULD INCREASE CONSUMPTION

Eating foods that are naturally rich in micronutrients is the secret to achieving optimal health and super immunity. A micronutrient-heavy diet supplies your body with 14 essential vitamins, 15 different minerals, and many thousands of phytochemicals, which are plant-based chemicals that have profound effects on human cell function and the immune system. Phytochemicals give plants their flavor, color and aroma. Foods that are naturally rich in these nutrients are also rich in fiber and water, and are naturally low in calories, meaning they have a low caloric density. These low-calorie, high-nutrient foods provide the ingredients that activate your body's self-healing and self-repairing mechanisms. The foundational principle of this program is that the right foods are your best medicine.

A poor diet is responsible for more deaths than any other risk factor worldwide (including smoking). The leading causes of death are heart disease and cancer, both of which are heavily influenced by what we eat.[1-3] In the early 20th century, when scientists first identified vitamins and minerals, they thought these nutrients could have a profound effect on reducing risks of cancer and other life-shortening diseases. Foods became fortified, and the supplement industry exploded. Vitamin-deficiency diseases plummeted; however, cancer rates increased. They realized vitamins and minerals alone were definitely not the answer.

Over time, we found out that the major micronutrient load in food was NOT vitamins and minerals; it was phytochemicals. Shockingly, natural foods contained many more critical nutritional elements than was ever imagined. There are thousands of micronutrients in fruits and vegetables, and when the right assortment of natural foods is consumed, these nutrients work harmoniously to increase our immunity and protect our body against disease.

The phytochemical revolution

All the different types of nutrients are vital to achieving and maintaining optimal health and nutritional excellence. However, phytochemicals hold a special, elite place in the nutritional landscape. When consistently consumed, in adequate quantity and variety, phytochemicals become super-nutrients in your body. They work together to detoxify cancer-causing compounds, deactivate free radicals, protect against radiation damage and enable DNA repair mechanisms.[4-6] When DNA defects are repaired, it can prevent cancer from developing later in life.

Consuming phytochemicals is not optional. They are essential in human immune-system defenses. Without a wide variety and sufficient number of phytochemicals from unprocessed plant foods, scientists note that cells age more rapidly and do not retain their innate ability to remove and detoxify waste products and toxic compounds. Low levels of phytochemical-rich produce in our modern diet is largely responsible for the common diseases seen with aging. The advances in modern nutritional science throughout this last decade can enable us to live longer and better, with almost no risk of the diseases that plague most Americans.

Let's take heart disease as an example. Heart attacks are extremely rare occurrences in populations that eat a diet rich in protective phytochemicals from vegetables, (such as the Kitavan islanders, even though most of them smoke cigarettes) but are omnipresent in populations, such as ours, that eat a diet low in these protective nutrients. Compelling data from numerous population studies shows that a natural, plant-based diet, rich in antioxidants and phytochemicals, will prevent, arrest, and even reverse heart disease.[7-13]

Our bodies were designed to make use of thousands of plant compounds. When these necessary compounds are missing, we survive because our bodies are adaptable; but over time, we lose our powerful potential for wellness, and chronic disease develops as we age. We suffer with physical, neurological, and emotional problems, become medically dependent, suffer needlessly and then die prematurely.

Eating right enables you to feel your best every day. You may still get sick from a virus, but your body will be in a far better position to defend itself and make a quick and complete recovery. Optimal nutrition enables us to work better, play better, and maintain our youthful vigor as we age gracefully.

The Health Equation

The secret to a long life and disease reversal is to eat a diet lower in calories but higher in nutrients. It is all about nutrient bang per caloric buck. This important nutritional concept can be presented by a simple mathematical formula, which I call my health equation.

DR. FUHRMAN'S HEALTH EQUATION:
H = N/C

Your Health is dependent on the Nutrient-per-Calorie density of your diet.

In this discussion, the word "nutrient" refers to micronutrients. This straightforward mathematical formula is the basis of nutritional science and nutritional healing. This formula essentially states that for you to be in excellent health, your diet must be nutrient-rich, and you must not overeat on calories (macronutrients). The nutrient density in your body's tissues is proportional to the nutrient density of your diet. You must seek out and consume more foods with a high nutrient-per-calorie density and fewer foods with a low nutrient-per-calorie density.

The most proven methodology to slow aging and extend human lifespan is moderate caloric restriction in the environment of micronutrient adequacy. This has been tested in every species of animal, including primates.[14] There is no controversy that Americans are eating themselves to death with too many calories. To change this we must do three things:

1 - EAT LESS FAT
2 - EAT LESS PROTEIN
3 - EAT LESS CARBOHYDRATE

Even though reduction of calories is valuable, the focus here is different. When the fatty foods you eat are high-nutrient fatty foods, and the proteins you eat are high-nutrient proteins, and the carbohydrates you eat are high-nutrient carbohydrates, you naturally desire fewer calories. Natural, whole plant foods are a mixture of fat, carbohydrate and protein, and in their natural state, they are typically rich in micronutrients. Simply trying to reduce calories is called dieting, and dieting doesn't work. The reason this program is so successful is because over time, without even trying or noticing it, you will prefer to eat fewer calories. I know that can sound unlikely. Many people think: "Not me" or "My body doesn't work that way" or "It will be a real struggle for me." However, if you follow the plan, it will happen instinctually and almost effortlessly. I have seen it happen to thousands of people, with all kinds of different backgrounds and eating histories. I promise, it can happen for you, too.

This program will help you achieve superior health and lose weight if you need to, by eating more nutrient-rich foods and fewer high-calorie, low-nutrient foods. It works because the more high-nutrient foods you consume, the less low-nutrient foods you desire. Foods are nutrient-dense when they contain a high level of micronutrients per calorie. Green vegetables win the award for the most nutrient-dense foods on the planet. Therefore, as you move forward in your quest for nutritional excellence, you will eat more and more vegetables. Since they contain the most nutrients per calorie, vegetables have the most powerful association with life extension and protection from heart disease and cancer.

It is also important to achieve micronutrient diversity. This means obtaining enough of all beneficial nutrients, not merely higher amounts of a select few. Eating a variety of plant foods is the key to achieving micronutrient diversity. Consider mushrooms and onions to illustrate this concept. They may not contain the highest amounts of vitamins and minerals, but they contain a significant amount of unique, protective phytochemicals that are not found in other foods.

Are You Making the Best Food Choices?

I have developed two different scoring systems to illustrate which foods are the highest in nutrient density. My **ANDI Scores** rate foods on a scale of 0-1000. ANDI is an easy way to visualize the relative nutrient value of various foods; it demonstrates the powerful differences between green vegetables and the foods that make up the biggest part of most people's diets. My **Nutrient IQ** is a new system that allows you to rate the nutritional quality of your daily diet by adding up points for the day to obtain a personalized nutrient score.

ANDI Scoring System

ANDI stands for Aggregate Nutrient Density Index. ANDI brings to life the H = N/C health equation or **Health = Nutrients** divided by **Calories** and shows you what foods you should eat to increase the micronutrient density of your diet. The "ANDI" Nutrient Score ranks foods on a scale of 0-1000 by assigning a score based on adding up the micronutrients they deliver for an equal-calorie serving. The most nutrient dense foods score 1000; all other foods are then scored relative to them. Kale, a dark leafy green, scores 1000, while Cola scores 0.6. Olive oil scores only 10 because it is high in calories and low in nutrients. This is an easy way to quickly visualize the relative nutrient value of various foods.

Using the ANDI is simple. It is meant to encourage you to eat more foods that have high numbers, and to eat larger amounts of these foods – because the higher the score, and the greater percentage of those foods in your diet, the better your health.

Test Your Nutrient IQ

How smart are you when it comes to making nutrient-dense food choices on a daily basis? You can find out by using my Nutrient IQ scoring system. It allows you to rate your diet each day, by adding up points for the day. Foods are assigned points based on their nutrient content and contribution to good health. You can adjust the points based on the size of the serving you eat.

As you might expect, the foods that have a high Nutrient IQ score are straight from nature – primarily vegetables, fruit and legumes – while refined, processed foods provide few or no points.

The Nutrient IQ point system differs from the ANDI (Aggregate Nutrient Density Index). While ANDI provides a ranking of foods based on the nutrients contained in an equal-calorie serving of each food, the Nutrient IQ Scores are connected to specific serving sizes of foods. This enables you to add up your scores and get a personal dietary rating each day.

Since the Nutrient IQ system is more closely tied to reasonable serving sizes, it provides a good estimate of the value of a food in your daily diet. For example, herbs such as parsley and basil have very high ANDI scores but since they are used only as seasonings, they may not contribute a great deal of nutrient value to your diet.

Nutrient IQ allows you to evaluate the quality of your diet and shows you how it can be improved. It demonstrates the nutritional value of colorful plants compared with that of animal products, oils, and processed foods. In case you haven't guessed, selecting a variety of vegetables, fruit and beans will provide the highest daily scores. Use these target scores to see how your diet measures up:

DAILY TARGET SCORES

	Men	Women
Good	700	600
Great	1000	800

Improving your daily score is about making better, more nutrient-dense food choices, not eating more food. To move up from Good to Great, you need to increase your servings of green leafy vegetables and cruciferous vegetables and make sure your daily menus include a well-rounded assortment of other high-Nutrient IQ vegetables, as well as beans, fruit, berries and seeds. Those who have a lower caloric need or are trying to lose weight may need to shoot for a lower Nutrient IQ score so they don't overeat when trying to increase their nutrients. Remember, more important than the total nutrients consumed is the nutrient-per-calorie density; so when you eat less, you need less nutrients.

Even though attention should be placed on nutrient-rich foods, it is also important to achieve micronutrient diversity and to eat an adequate assortment of moderately-ranked plant foods in order to obtain the full range of human dietary requirements. Include some Greens, Beans, Onions, Mushrooms, Berries and Seeds in your diet every day. Think G-BOMBS!

The serving sizes listed in the table below and in Chapter Six are convenient measurements; they are not necessarily recommended serving amounts. Adjust your scores based on the amount of the food that you eat. For example, the table lists 90 points for 1 cup of broccoli, so if you have 2 cups, give yourself 180 points. If a medium tomato is worth 60 points, then give yourself 30 points for eating half. If a vegetable, fruit, bean or whole grain food you are looking for is not listed in the table, assign it a value based on a similar food item. Assume that most processed, refined foods and anything made with refined white flour and white sugar provide zero points.

Please note that you do NOT have to score foods and keep track of points to eat a Nutritarian diet and be healthy. You do not have to keep track of your calories. These scoring systems are motivational tools to help you to learn how to eat more healthfully. You only need to understand how to lay out a healthful and nutritionally balanced menu, and then stick to it.

Matter of Emphasis

Most health authorities today are in agreement that we should add more servings of healthy fruits and vegetables to our diet. I disagree. Thinking about our diet in this fashion doesn't adequately address the problem. Instead of adding those protective fruits, vegetables, beans, seeds and nuts to our disease-causing diet, these foods must be the main focus of the diet itself. This is what makes the Nutritarian approach different.

The following chart provides a sample of ANDI and Nutrient IQ scores for several different foods. Please refer to Chapter Six for additional scores.

Since phytochemicals are largely unnamed and unmeasured, these rankings may actually underestimate the healthful properties of colorful, natural plant foods, so the comparative nutrient density of many of these whole foods may be even higher than the scores indicate.

SAMPLE ANDI AND NUTRIENT IQ SCORES

	ANDI	Nutrient IQ (serving size)
Kale, cooked	1000	112 (1 cup)
Bok Choy	865	90 (1 cup)
Broccoli	340	90 (1 cup)
Romaine	510	64 (2 cups)
Tomato	186	60 (1 medium)
Mushrooms	238	60 (1/4 cup)
Onions, raw	32	60 (1/4 cup)
Black Beans	61	52 (1/2 cup)
Carrots	458	45 (1 cup)
Corn	45	45 (1 cup)
Strawberries	182	45 (1/2 cup)
Flax Seeds	103	41 (1 tablespoon)
Quinoa	28	26 (1 cup)
White Potato	28	12 (1 medium)
Salmon	34	7 (4 ounces)

CHAPTER FOUR

TWO LEVELS OF
SUPERIOR NUTRITION

Based on your health needs and current dietary habits, you can choose between two levels of superior nutrition:

Level One: Good
Level Two: Great

I would like to see everyone reach Level One. For many, even Level One represents a significant improvement. In addition, some people do better by starting with Level One and gradually reaching Level Two. However, if you are overweight, struggle with food addictions, suffer from a medical condition or want to strive for maximum longevity, you should move as quickly as possible to Level Two.

Use the ANDI and Nutrient IQ scores contained in Chapter Six of this book to help you choose the most nutrient-dense foods and to tally your daily intake. As you learn more about eating this way, you will begin to understand that increasing your green-vegetable consumption pumps up your degree of nutritional excellence. Green vegetables are the most micronutrient-rich-per-calorie foods. You will find sample menus and healthy recipes in Chapters Seven and Eight. Nutrient-dense soups, smoothies, dressings, dips, entrees and desserts are featured in all the meal plans contained in my books and website, www. DrFuhrman.com. For a greater understanding of the Nutritarian diet, I suggest reading my latest book, *Eat for Life*.

No matter which level you choose, take a 28-day Nutritarian Pledge to follow these cornerstones of healthy eating:

Include daily:
1. A large salad (in a 9 oz. bowl, not a 6 oz. one)
2. At least a half-cup serving of beans/legumes in soup, salad or a main dish
3. At least three fresh fruits
4. One ounce or 1/4 cup of raw nuts and seeds, with half being walnuts, or chia, hemp, flax or sesame seeds. If trying to lose weight, limit to 1.5 ounces for women and 2 ounces for men
5. At least one large (double-size) serving of steamed green vegetables
6. 1/4 cup raw onion
7. 1/4 cup cooked mushrooms

Avoid:
1. Barbecued, processed and red meat
2. Fried foods
3. Dairy (cheese, ice cream, butter, whole milk and 2% milk)
4. Soft drinks, sugar and other sweetening agents or artificial sweeteners
5. White flour products
6. Oil
7. Salt

The point is to give your body a real chance to change its biochemistry and build up its nutrient stores. You will see how much better your life can be when you are well nourished.

Level 1: Good (Men: 700 IQ points, Women: 600 IQ points)

Level 1 is appropriate for a person who is healthy, thin, physically fit and exercises regularly. You should have no risk factors such as high blood pressure, high cholesterol or a family history of heart disease, stroke or cancer before the age of 75.

You can significantly revamp your diet at this level. Enjoy this new style of eating, allow your taste preferences to change with time, and try some great recipes.

The majority of individuals, however, should make the

commitment to move quickly to Level 2 or jump right into this more nutrient-dense level, because so many people are significantly overweight and have risk factors that need to be addressed immediately. People in desperate need of a health makeover need to start on Level 2.

Having superior nutrition is key to having optimal health. That's because when you incorporate more and more nutrient-rich produce in your diet, you automatically increase your intake of antioxidants, phytochemicals, plant fibers, and plant sterols. You lower the glycemic index of your diet and the level of saturated fat, salt and other negative elements without having to think about it. Your ability to appreciate the natural flavors of unprocessed, whole foods improves with time as your taste buds increase their sensitivity, once added salt and sugar no longer overwhelm them.

Steps to implement now:

1. Add more beans and nuts to your diet to replace animal products.

2. Eliminate fried foods and water sauté instead.

3. Avoid commercial baked goods and sweetened desserts and instead substitute fruit-based desserts, such as frozen "nice" creams, bean-based brownies and avocado chocolate pudding, to name a few. You'll be pleasantly surprised at how delicious they are – and knowing that

they're actually good for you increases your enjoyment of them.

4. Use intact, whole grain products like millet, quinoa, buckwheat, teff, farro and rolled or steel-cut oats. Replace white flour pasta with the many different types that are more nutrient-dense, such as bean, chickpea and cauliflower pastas.

5. Use only a minimal amount of oil. Try some of the high-nutrient dressing and dip recipes in Chapter Eight. They use heart-healthy nuts and seeds to replace the oils found in traditional dressings, sauces and dips.

6. Eliminate foods like cheese and butter, which are high in saturated fats, and egg yolks, which are high in cholesterol. In Level 1, I recommend only three small servings of animal products per week. These animal products are limited to egg whites, fat-free dairy, wild fish and certified organic poultry. Most Americans consume over 20 servings of animal products weekly. Plant-based foods including nuts, seeds, beans, and bean products like tofu, tempeh, and bean pasta are used to replace animal products.

Your sodium intake will decrease as you begin to make these dietary changes. Aside from the sodium naturally present in whole plants, limit your additional sodium intake to 500mg if you are at Level 1 and to 300mg at Level 2. Processed foods and restaurant foods contribute 71%

of the sodium people consume. Salt from the saltshaker provides 11%, and sodium found naturally in food provides about 14% of the amount people consume.[1]

How much you should eat varies widely from person to person, but if you are not at your ideal weight, you should be moving closer to achieving it every day. If you are significantly overweight or obese, you should be losing at least two pounds a week on your way to recovery. You will find that the better you adhere to a nutrient-dense, plant-rich diet style, the more your hunger sensations are transformed, and you simply desire fewer calories.

Level 2: Great (Men: 1000 IQ points, Women: 800 IQ points)

If you suffer from a serious medical condition, such as diabetes, heart disease, or autoimmune disease, or just want to optimize the nutrient density of your diet to slow aging and maximize longevity, step up to or start at Level 2. If you suffer from a medical condition that is important to reverse or are on medications and you want to be able to discontinue them as quickly as possible, Level 2 is the right prescription. It is also the level to choose if you have trouble losing weight no matter what you do, and want to maximize your results.

Level 2 is the diet that I use in my medical practice for people who have some type of serious condition, such as autoimmune disease (e.g. rheumatoid arthritis or lupus), heart disease, diabetes (type 1 or type 2), migraines, or gastro-intestinal problems. For people who are post-cancer, have cancer or are at high risk of getting cancer, I prescribe

Level 2 with the added stipulation of zero animal products. Level 2 delivers the highest level of nutrient density. It is the level I eat.

A maximum of two small servings (each serving smaller than a deck of cards) of animal products weekly is allowed on Level 2, if a person chooses not to be vegan. I am all for being vegan and frequently prescribe it, but for many people it is not essential.

Level 2 maximizes vegetable consumption. Use green smoothies, fresh vegetable juices, healthful soups and lots of cooked greens and raw vegetables to make every calorie count. Use the Nutrient IQ scores in Chapter Six to select the most nutrient-dense foods possible.

At this level, you should consume processed foods only rarely. Keep the use of refined fats and oils to a minimum. Nuts and seeds supply essential fats in a much healthier package, with significant health benefits. The menus and recipes in Chapters Seven and Eight provide some ideas for incorporating a variety of nutrient dense foods into your diet.

In the following table, I have listed some of the top foods in the six food categories that should make up 75-80% of your diet. These foods get some of the highest Nutrient IQ scores. Below each group is listed the number of daily servings suggested to achieve Level 1 or 2. These amounts should not be seen as rigid requirements, but rather as helpful guidelines. Of course, there are many other choices in these categories, and I encourage you to try them all.

Two Levels of Superior Nutrition

Recommended Servings of Vegetables, Fruit, Beans and Nuts

COOKED GREEN VEGETABLES

1½ cups kale

1 ½ cups mustard, turnip
or collard greens

1 ½ cups Bok choy

1 ½ cups broccoli rabe

1 ½ cups cabbage

1 ½ cups spinach

1 ½ cups Brussels sprouts

1 ½ cups Swiss chard

1 ½ cups broccoli

LEVEL ONE	LEVEL TWO
1-2 servings	2-3 servings

RAW GREEN VEGETABLES

3 cups watercress

5 cups spinach

5 cups romaine, Boston,
red or green leaf lettuce

5 cups arugula

5 cups mixed baby greens

½ cups raw broccoli

½ cups cabbage

½ cups green pepper

2 cups zucchini

½ cups snow peas

LEVEL ONE	LEVEL TWO
2-3 servings	3-4 servings

NON-GREEN VEGETABLES

1 cup carrots

6 radishes

1 cup red pepper

2 cups radicchio

1 cup cauliflower

1 tomato

1/2 cup chopped onion or scallions

1/2 cup cooked mushrooms

LEVEL ONE
1-2 servings

LEVEL TWO
2-3 servings

FRUIT

1 ½ cups strawberries

1 ½ cups raspberries

1 ½ cups blueberries

2 plums

1 orange

1 ½ cups cantaloupe

2 kiwis

2 ½ cups watermelon

1 apple

1 ½ cups cherries

LEVEL ONE
3-5 servings

LEVEL TWO
3-5 servings

BEANS

½ - 1 cup lentils

½ - 1 cup red kidney

½ - 1 cup black beans

½ - 1 cup pinto beans

½ - 1 cup split peas

½ - 1 cup edamame

½ - 1 cup chickpeas

½ - 1 cup white beans

1 cup cooked bean pasta

4 oz tempeh

LEVEL ONE
1-3 servings

LEVEL TWO
1-3 servings

NUTS AND SEEDS

1/4 cup sunflower seeds

2 tablespoons ground flax, hemp or chia seeds

2 tablespoons sesame seeds

1/4 cup pumpkin seeds

1/4 cup walnuts

1/4 cup pistachios

1/4 cup pecans

1/4 cup almonds

1/4 cup cashews

2 tablespoons raw nut or seed butter

LEVEL ONE
1-3 servings*

LEVEL TWO
1-3 servings*

The amount of nuts and seeds, as well as other foods you consume, depends on your caloric requirements. If you are trying to lose weight, limit nuts to one serving daily. If you are thin, want to gain weight or need more calories to fuel your athletic activities, then the number of servings may be increased.

Eating enough healthy food is critical to your success as a Nutritarian. You will find that when you eat enough high-nutrient food, you no longer desire – or even have room for – the other foods that used to make up the biggest part of your diet. Processed and refined foods offer little in terms of nutrients and phytochemicals. When you eat them, you are literally throwing away valuable nutrients that could have been put to good use by your body.

Overview of Two Levels – Recommended Amounts

	LEVEL 1 (GOOD)	LEVEL 2 (GREAT)
	Target Nutrient IQ points: Men – 700 / Women - 600	Target Nutrient IQ points: Men – 1000 / Women - 800
Vegetables raw & cooked 1 serving = 1 ½ cups cooked or 2 to 5 cups raw	4-7 servings /day	7-10 servings /day
Fruit 1 serving = about 1 ½ cups	3-5 servings /day	3-5 servings /day
Beans 1 serving = ½ to 1 cup	1-2 servings /day	1-2 servings /day
Nuts & Seeds 1 serving = 1 ounce or ¼ cup Limit to 1 serving if trying to lose weight	1-3 servings /day	1-3 servings /day
Whole Grain Products/ Potatoes 1 serving = 1 slice or 1 cup	1-2 servings /day	1-2 servings /day
Animal Products* 1 serving = 2 ounce	3 servings/week or less	2 servings/week or less
Sodium	1200 mg/day or less	1000 mg/day or less
Fats/Oils* Avoid processed, refined fats and oil. A small amount of olive oil may be used if you are not trying to lose weight.	maximum of 2 tablespoons of olive oil/week	maximum of 1 tablespoon of olive oil/week

*If you are overweight and/or struggle with food addictions and cravings, avoid animal products and oil entirely. They can trigger overeating behavior.

1. U.S. Centers for Disease Control and Prevention: Sodium and Food Sources [https://www.cdc.gov/salt/food.html]

CHAPTER FIVE

TOP NUTRITARIAN PRINCIPLES

Here is my Top Ten list of Nutritarian principles.

1. Your body's immune system needs the right foods to allow it to work to its fullest potential.

By changing our diet and combining foods that contain powerful immune-strengthening capabilities, we can achieve incredible health and prevent and even reverse disease. The standard American diet is deficient in nutrients. We are eating too many highly processed foods, foods with added sweeteners, foods with animal fats and animal proteins. At the same time, we are not eating enough fruits, vegetables, seeds and beans, which leaves us lacking in hundreds of the most immune-building compounds.

2. Dr. Fuhrman's Health Equation: H=N/C

Your long-term **Health** is directly related to the amount of **Nutrients** you get for each **Calorie**. The more nutrient-dense your diet is, the more disease protection you earn. The most nutrient-dense foods are fruits and vegetables – especially dark leafy greens, which are the foods missing in most modern diets. Nutrient-dense foods contain vital nutrients, vitamins and minerals essential for preventing disease, boosting immunity, detoxifying your body and delivering permanent weight loss.

3. Prescription medications will not solve your health problems.

Heart disease, Type II diabetes, hypertension and many other conditions are directly related to poor dietary habits. The body has an incredible ability to heal itself when properly nourished. For example, even patients on insulin for years can reduce, and eventually eliminate medications as they lose weight and become healthy. Superior nutrition is more effective than medications at resolving most medical problems while promoting a pleasurable, longer and more healthful life.

4. If you want to lose weight — DON'T DIET!

Most of the weight lost on popular diets is regained. While many diets may produce short term weight loss, they cannot be maintained, and therefore, the weight returns. The only proven strategy for permanent weight loss is to consume sufficient nutrients and fiber for a lifetime of excellent health. This strategy will reduce your cravings for "junk'" food, and curb the tendency to overeat. You will instinctually eat fewer calories, without the food addiction and cravings that have sabotaged your attempts in the past.

5. Where's the Beef?

Remember that vegetables, beans and seeds are high in protein, so there is no essential need to eat animal products for protein. Think about it: Cows are vegan, as are gorillas and horses. Are you trying to lose weight or reduce your cholesterol? Think greens for health and for building lean muscle. To maximize our health and longevity, we need to get more protein from nutrient-rich plant sources such as greens, beans, seeds, and nuts – and less from animal products.

6. Remember: G-BOMBS

Greens, Beans, Onions, Mushrooms, Berries and Seeds are important foods with powerful immune-strengthening capabilities. Include these super foods in your diet every day.

7. Watch the Olive Oil!

One tablespoon of olive oil has 120 calories (all oils do).

One-quarter cup has 500 calories. Healthy salads are a way of life for people who want to lose weight or improve health. However, many of the benefits of a salad are lost when the calorie count is increased ten-fold with refined oil. Nut and seed-based dressings are the way to go. Nuts and seeds, not oil, have shown dramatic protection against heart disease. We need to get more of our fats from these wholesome foods and less from processed oils.

8. If health came in a bottle, we'd all be healthy!

Natural, whole, plant-based foods are highly complex. It may never be possible to extract the precise symphony of nutrients found in fruits and vegetables and place it in a pill. So don't rely on pills and supplements to get your primary nutrition.

9. Six-A-Day – Not the Way!

You have probably heard it's better to eat six small meals a day. That is not ideal. You simply will not need to eat that frequently once your body is well nourished with micronutrients. The body can more effectively detoxify and enhance cell repair when it is not constantly eating and digesting. Eating healthfully removes cravings and reduces the sensations that drive us to eat too much and too often. For most people who follow a Nutritarian diet, eating when truly hungry means eating three, or maybe two meals a day.

10. Let Your Body Decide!

Nobody wants to hear that they must give up all their favorite foods, such as pizza and ice cream. But wouldn't it be nice if, over time, your body actually preferred healthy foods? The body can change its taste and food preferences. As you consume larger and larger portions of health-promoting foods, your appetite for low-nutrient foods decreases, and you gradually lose your addiction to sugar and fats. You learn to enjoy and prepare gourmet-tasting meals that are nutrient-rich. When this occurs, you have become a Nutritarian!

I realize unhealthy foods can be very appealing and hard to resist. Please be patient with yourself as you start to eat right. As you switch to healthful foods, you will lose your cravings for unhealthful foods. You will learn to eat only when you are truly hungry. Your body will learn to love fresh fruits and vegetables and my healthful recipes because they taste so great and satisfying.

Becoming a Nutritarian is all about having the knowledge and support you need to get back in touch with the natural wisdom of your body.

CHAPTER SIX

NUTRIENT IQ
AND ANDI SCORES

	CALORIES	SODIUM (mg)	NUT. IQ	ANDI

VEGETABLES

	CALORIES	SODIUM (mg)	NUT. IQ	ANDI
Kale, cooked (1 cup)	43	19	112	1000
Mustard greens, cooked (1 cup)	36	13	112	1000
Collard greens, cooked (1 cup)	63	29	112	1000
Turnip greens, cooked (1 cup)	29	42	112	1000
Watercress, cooked (1 cup)	15	247	112	1000
Swiss chard, cooked (1 cup)	35	313	112	895
Bok choy, raw (1 cup)	9	46	90	865
Bok choy, cooked (1 cup)	20	58	90	865
Radishes, raw (1 cup)	19	45	90	502
Brussels sprouts, raw (1 cup)	38	22	90	490

	CALORIES	SODIUM (mg)	NUT. IQ	ANDI
Brussels sprouts, cooked (1 cup)	56	33	90	490
Turnips, raw (1 cup)	36	87	90	473
Turnips, cooked (1 cup)	34	25	90	473
Cabbage, cooked (1 cup) (green, red, napa, savoy)	34	12	90	434
Broccoli rabe, raw (1 cup)	9	13	90	366
Broccoli rabe, cooked (1 cup)	43	95	90	366
Kohlrabi, raw (1 cup)	36	27	90	352
Kohlrabi, cooked (1 cup)	48	35	90	352
Broccoli, raw (1 cup)	31	30	90	340
Cauliflower, raw (1 cup)	27	32	90	315
Broccoli, cooked (1 cup)	55	64	90	294
Cauliflower, cooked (1 cup)	29	32	90	294
Spinach, cooked (1 cup)	41	126	82	707
Escarole, cooked (1 cup)	23	29	82	516
Endive, cooked (1 cup)	23	29	82	284
Kale, raw (1 cup)	7	11	79	778
Mustard greens, raw (1 cup)	15	11	79	1000
Collard greens, raw (1 cup)	12	6	79	1000
Turnip greens, raw (1 cup)	18	22	79	1000
Swiss chard, raw (1 cup)	7	77	79	1000
Watercress, raw (1 cup)	4	14	79	1000
Arugula, raw (1 cup)	5	5	79	604
Cabbage, raw, (1 cup) (green, red, napa, savoy)	22	16	79	332

	CALORIES	SODIUM (mg)	NUT. IQ	ANDI
Spinach, raw (2 cups)	14	47	64	705
Mixed baby greens (2 cups)	12	20	64	585
Escarole, raw (2 cups)	13	18	64	516
Romaine lettuce (2 cups)	13	18	64	510
Red or green leaf lettuce (2 cups)	14	14	64	507
Boston or Bibb lettuce (2 cups)	7	3	64	367
Endive, raw (2 cups)	9	11	64	284
Fennel, raw (1 cup)	27	45	64	284
Green pepper, raw (1 cup)	18	3	64	207
Asparagus, raw (1 cup)	27	3	64	205
Asparagus, cooked (1 cup)	40	25	64	205
Zucchini, cooked (1 cup)	27	5	64	164
Green pepper, cooked (1 cup)	38	3	64	158
Okra, cooked (1 cup)	35	10	64	155
Artichokes (1 item)	64	120	64	145
Artichokes (3/4 cup hearts)	67	108	64	145
Zucchini, raw (1 cup)	21	10	64	142
Snow peas, raw (1 cup)	27	3	64	106
Sugar snap peas, raw (1 cup)	27	3	64	99
Green beans, raw (1 cup)	31	6	64	99
Snow peas, cooked (1 cup)	67	6	64	97
Cucumber (1 cup)	17	3	64	87
Green beans, cooked (1 cup)	44	1	64	81
Sugar snap peas, cooked (1 cup)	67	6	64	81

	CALORIES	SODIUM (mg)	NUT. IQ	ANDI
Radicchio, raw (1 cup)	9	9	60	271
Red Pepper, cooked (1 cup)	38	1	60	265
Tomato sauce, no salt added (1 cup)	78	37	60	244
Red pepper, raw (1 cup)	39	6	60	224
Mushrooms, cooked (1/4 cup)	11	1	60	238
Tomatoes, raw (1 cup or 1 medium tomato)	32	9	60	186
Tomatoes, cooked (1 cup)	43	26	60	184
Bean sprouts, raw (1 cup)	31	6	60	177
Bean sprouts, cooked (1 cup)	62	11	60	177
Tomato paste (1 tablespoon)	13	9	60	174
Pasta sauce, low sodium (1 cup)	131	77	60	137
Leeks, raw (1/4 cup)	14	5	60	135
Garlic, raw (1/4 cup)	51	6	60	118
Garlic, raw (1 clove)	5	1	5	118
Onions, raw (1/4 cup)	16	2	60	107
Shallots, raw (1/4 cup)	29	1	60	107
Scallions/green onions, raw (1/4 cup)	8	4	60	94
Yellow squash, cooked (1 cup)	36	2	60	92
Yellow squash, raw (1 cup)	18	2	60	88
Eggplant, cooked (1 cup)	35	1	60	31
Carrots, cooked (1 cup)	55	45	45	458
Carrots, raw (1 cup)	53	88	45	384
Carrots, raw (1 medium)	25	42	23	384
Rutabaga, cooked (1 cup)	51	9	45	296

	CALORIES	SODIUM (mg)	NUT. IQ	ANDI
Pumpkin, cooked (1 cup)	49	2	45	249
Butternut squash, cooked (1 cup)	82	8	45	241
Potato, sweet, cooked (1 cup or 1 medium)	180	72	45	181
Beets, raw (1 cup)	59	106	45	80
Green peas, cooked (1 cup)	134	5	45	63
Beets, cooked (1 cup)	75	65	45	57
Corn, cooked (1 cup)	143	1	45	45
Acorn squash, cooked (1 cup)	115	8	45	44
Spaghetti squash, cooked (1 cup)	42	28	45	44
Parsnips, cooked (1 cup)	55	8	45	37
Leeks, cooked (1/4 cup)	8	3	30	135
Garlic, cooked (1/4 cup)	49	21	30	118
Onions, shallots and green onions, cooked (1/4 cup)	23	6	30	109
Salsa, no-salt-added (1/4 cup)	19	4	26	179
Turmeric, ground (1 teaspoon)	9	1	25	298
Turmeric, fresh, chopped (1 tablespoon)	24	0	25	298
Avocado (1/4 cup or ¼ avocado)	60	3	23	28
Potato, white, cooked (1 cup or 1 medium)	113	6	12	28
Celery, raw (1/2 cup)	7	81	11	151
Celery, cooked (1/2 cup)	27	136	11	151
Iceberg lettuce (2 cups)	16	11	11	127
Basil, fresh, chopped (2 tablespoons)	1	0	10	518

	CALORIES	SODIUM (mg)	NUT. IQ	ANDI
Cilantro, fresh, chopped (2 tablespoons)	1	1	10	481
Cinnamon, ground (1 teaspoon)	6	0	10	426
Dill, fresh, chopped (2 tablespoons)	1	0	10	381
Parsley, fresh, chopped (2 tablespoons)	3	4	10	381
Ginger Root, fresh, chopped (1 tablespoon)	10	1	10	56

FRUIT

	CALORIES	SODIUM (mg)	NUT. IQ	ANDI
Cranberries, fresh not dried (1/2 cup)	23	1	45	207
Strawberries (1/2 cup)	27	2	45	182
Blueberries (1/2 cup)	42	1	45	132
Raspberries (1/2 cup)	32	1	45	133
Blackberries (1/2 cup)	31	1	45	132
Goji berries, dried (1/2 cup)	156	133	45	120
Gooseberries (1/2 cup)	33	1	45	111
Cherries (2/3 cup)	43	0	41	85
Pomegranate kernels (1/4 cup)	36	1	37	119
Pomegranate juice (1/4 cup)	34	6	37	102
Grapefruit (1 cup or ½ grapefruit)	76	0	19	120
Grapes (1 cup)	104	3	19	119
Cantaloupe (1 cup)	54	26	19	118
Plums (1 cup or 2 items)	61	0	19	106
Oranges (3/4 cup peeled sections or 1 medium)	62	0	19	98

	CALORIES	SODIUM (mg)	NUT. IQ	ANDI
Mandarin oranges (3/4 cup peeled sections or 2 items)	77	3	19	91
Clementines (3/4 cup peeled sections or 2 items)	70	1	19	91
Tangerines (3/4 cup peeled sections or 2 items)	77	3	19	86
Apricots, fresh (1 cup or 2 items)	34	0	19	75
Watermelon (1 cup)	46	2	19	71
Papaya (1 cup)	62	12	19	69
Peaches (1 cup or 1 item)	60	0	19	65
Kiwi (1 cup or 2 items)	84	4	19	61
Figs, fresh (2 figs)	74	1	19	56
Pineapple (1 cup)	83	2	19	54
Mango (1 cup or ½ mango)	99	2	19	53
Kumquats (4 items)	54	8	19	51
Pears (1 cup or 1 item)	101	2	19	40
Honeydew (1 cup)	61	31	19	31
Nectarines (1 cup or 1 item)	63	0	19	39
Coconut, fresh (1 cup)	283	16	19	14
Apple (1 cup or 1 item)	95	2	11	53
Banana (1 cup or 1 item)	105	1	11	30

	CALORIES	SODIUM (mg)	NUT. IQ	ANDI

DRIED FRUIT

	CALORIES	SODIUM (mg)	NUT. IQ	ANDI
Blueberries, dried, unsweetened (1/4 cup)	129	1	8	74
Cherries, dried, unsweetened (1/4 cup)	118	24	8	44
Figs (1/4 cup)	93	4	5	56
Figs (1 fig)	21	1	2	56
Apricots (1/4 cup)	78	3	5	26
Currants (1/4 cup)	102	3	5	21
Dates, (1/4 cup)	104	1	5	17
Dates (1 medjool date)	67	0	3	17
Dates (1 deglet noor date)	20	0	1	17
Raisins (1/4 cup)	109	4	5	15
Coconut, dried, unsweetened (1/4 cup)	139	8	5	10
Cranberries, dried, sweetened (1/4 cup)	85	1	0	42

BEANS

	CALORIES	SODIUM (mg)	NUT. IQ	ANDI
Edamame (1/2 cup)	65	3	52	98
Navy, cooked (1/2 cup)	128	0	52	77
Cannellini, cooked (1/2 cup)	113	1	52	77
Lentils, cooked (1/2 cup)	115	2	52	72
Lima beans (1/2 cup)	108	2	52	69
Kidney, cooked (1/2 cup)	113	1	52	64
Black, cooked (1/2 cup)	114	1	52	61
Chickpeas, cooked (1/2 cup)	135	6	52	55

	CALORIES	SODIUM (mg)	NUT. IQ	ANDI
Bean pasta, cooked (1 cup)	200	0	52	50
Bean pasta, dry (2 ounces)	200	0	52	50
Split peas, cooked (1/2 cup)	116	2	52	43
Tempeh (1 cup)	319	15	45	66
Hummus (1/4 cup)	146	149	35	47
Tofu (1 cup)	362	35	15	82
Soy milk (1 cup)	105	115	15	37

NUTS AND SEEDS

(VALUES FOR SODIUM ARE FOR NO-SALT-ADDED
NUTS, SEEDS AND NUT AND SEED BUTTERS)

	CALORIES	SODIUM (mg)	NUT. IQ	ANDI
Walnuts (1/4 cup)	164	0	45	30
Flax seeds (2 tablespoons)	112	6	41	103
Chia seeds (2 tablespoons)	99	3	41	77
Hemp seeds (2 tablespoons)	111	1	41	65
Sunflower seeds (1/4 cup)	204	3	34	64
Sesame seeds (1/4 cup)	206	4	34	56
Pumpkin seeds (1/4 cup)	180	2	34	39
Pistachio nuts (1/4 cup)	172	0	26	37
Hazelnuts (1/4 cup)	212	0	26	34
Pecans (1/4 cup)	171	0	26	33
Almonds (1/4 cup)	206	0	26	28
Pine nuts (1/4 cup)	227	1	26	28
Cashews (1/4 cup)	188	4	26	27
Brazil nuts (1/4 cup)	219	1	26	26
Hemp milk, unsweetened (1 cup)	60	110	15	30

	CALORIES	SODIUM (mg)	NUT. IQ	ANDI
Almond milk, unsweetened (1 cup)	37	173	15	26
Coconut milk, unsweetened (1 cup)	45	70	15	26
Macadamia nuts (1/4 cup)	240	2	15	21
Tahini (1 tablespoon)	89	5	13	60
Sunflower butter (1 tablespoon)	99	0	13	55
Almond butter (1 tablespoon)	98	1	13	29
Cashew butter (1 tablespoon)	94	2	13	26
Peanuts, unsalted (1/4 cup)	219	2	11	59
Peanut butter, low sodium (1 tablespoon)	96	3	6	51

GRAINS

WHOLE GRAINS

Wild rice, cooked (1 cup)	101	3	26	56
Wild rice, dry (1/4 cup)	143	3	26	56
Teff, cooked (1 cup)	255	20	26	46
Steel cut oats, cooked (1 cup)	166	0	26	36
Steel cut oats, dry (1/4 cup)	150	0	26	36
Bulgar, cooked (1 cup)	151	9	26	33
Buckwheat, cooked (1 cup)	155	7	26	30
Buckwheat, dry (1/4 cup)	146	2	26	30
Farro, cooked (1 cup)	200	0	26	30
Farro, dry (1/3 cup)	211	0	26	30
Quinoa, cooked (1 cup)	222	13	26	28
Quinoa, dry (1/3 cup)	209	2	26	28

	CALORIES	SODIUM (mg)	NUT. IQ	ANDI
Barley, cooked (1 cup)	198	5	26	24
Barley, dry (1/3 cup)	217	7	26	24
Old fashioned oats, cooked (1 cup)	166	0	19	36
Old fashioned oats, dry (1/2 cup)	150	0	19	36
Cornmeal, dry(1/4 cup)	111	43	11	17
Bread, 100% whole grain (1 slice)	80	80	7	30
Brown rice, cooked (1 cup)	248	8	7	28
Brown rice, uncooked (1/4 cup)	170	2	7	28
Pita, 100% whole grain (1 item)	90	110	7	26
Wraps, 100% whole grain (1 item)	150	140	7	24

REFINED GRAIN PRODUCTS

(NUMBERS IN PARENTHESIS ARE ESTIMATES OF WHAT SCORE WOULD BE WITH-OUT FORTIFICATION. SEE PAGE 71 FOR NOTE ON FORTIFICATION)

	CALORIES	SODIUM (mg)	NUT. IQ	ANDI
Cold cereals (1 cup) made from 100% whole grains and nuts without added sweeteners	varies	varies	11	67 (26)
Cold cereals, not 100% whole grain	varies	varies	0	54 (3)
Pasta, whole wheat, cooked (1 cup)	186	7	7	25 (22)
Pasta, white, cooked (1 cup)	190	1	0	16 (11)
Quick oats, cooked (1 cup)	166	9	4	21
Instant oats, cooked (1 cup)	230	266	4	21
Couscous, cooked (1 cup)	176	8	0	13 (10)
Whole wheat bread products, not 100% whole wheat bread, wraps, pita, bagels	varies	varies	0	19-21
White bread products, all refined white flour bread, wraps, pita, bagels	varies	varies	0	12 (5)-17 (9)
Crackers	varies	varies	0	11 (5)

DAIRY PRODUCTS AND EGGS

	CALORIES	SODIUM (mg)	NUT. IQ	ANDI
Eggs (1 item)	72	71	4	31
Milk, skim (1 cup)	83	102	4	38
Milk, 1% (1 cup)	102	107	4	31
Milk, 2% (1 cup)	122	115	3	27
Milk, whole (1 cup)	149	105	3	22
Plain Yogurt, fat free and low fat, no added sugar (6 ounces)	varies	varies	4	28-33
Plain Yogurt, full fat, no added sugar (6 ounces)	varies	varies	3	20
Yogurt with added sugar	varies	varies	0	15
Frozen yogurt	varies	varies	0	18
Cottage cheese (1 cup)	185	706	2	21
Feta cheese (2 ounces)	150	633	2	20
Cream cheese (2 ounces)	194	182	2	6
Cream cheese, low fat (2 ounces)	115	268	2	11
All other cheeses	varies	varies	2	11-16
Ice cream	varies	varies	0	6-9

	CALORIES	SODIUM (mg)	NUT. IQ	ANDI

FISH

	CALORIES	SODIUM (mg)	NUT. IQ	ANDI
Wild salmon (4 ounces)	207	63	7	34
Farmed salmon (4 ounces)	233	69	5	34
Lower mercury fish (4 ounces) sole, flounder, cod, bass, haddock, hake, sardine, trout, squid, catfish, tilapia, mackerel, squid	varies	varies	5	25-33
All other seafood (4 ounces) such as tuna, halibut, red snapper, swordfish, grouper mahi mahi, orange roughy, shark	varies	varies	4	23-30

SHELLFISH

	CALORIES	SODIUM (mg)	NUT. IQ	ANDI
Oysters (6 items)	43	71	5	139
Lobster, boiled (4 ounces)	101	551	5	67
Crab, boiled (4 ounces)	94	448	5	60
Mussels (4 ounces)	194	417	5	60
Shrimp, boiled (4 ounces)	112	126	5	42
Clams (6 items)	75	523	5	26

	CALORIES	SODIUM (mg)	NUT. IQ	ANDI

POULTRY

	CALORIES	SODIUM (mg)	NUT. IQ	ANDI
Ground Turkey, 93% Lean, broiled (4 ounces)	235	103	4	26
Turkey breast, roasted, (4 ounces)	178	73	4	24
Chicken breast, roasted (4 ounces)	196	87	4	24
Chicken, dark meat, roasted (4 ounces)	232	105	4	18
Italian-style turkey sausage (4 ounces)	179	1052	0	26
Chicken nuggets (4 ounces)	336	632	0	11
Turkey bacon, cooked (2 ounces)	214	1280	0	10
Turkey hot dog, 1 item	100	485	0	14

OTHER MEAT

	CALORIES	SODIUM (mg)	NUT. IQ	ANDI
Beef, all varieties	varies	varies	0	14-26
Pork, all varieties	varies	varies	0	14-29
Lamb, all varieties	varies	varies	0	17-21
Ham, cured, roasted (4 ounces)	275	1345	0	17
Bacon, cooked (2 ounces)	307	1310	0	13
Italian-style pork sausage (4 ounces)	390	1369	0	13
Pepperoni, (2 ounces)	277	926	0	12
Beef and pork hot dog, 1 item	137	504	0	10
Breakfast sausage (4 ounces)	363	1034	0	7

	CALORIES	SODIUM (mg)	NUT. IQ	ANDI

DESSERT ITEMS

	CALORIES	SODIUM (mg)	NUT. IQ	ANDI
Cocoa Powder, unsweetened (2 tablespoons)	24	2	7	130
Dark chocolate, 80-100% cocoa (1.5 ounces)	255	9	7	54
Dark chocolate, 65-79% cocoa (1.5 ounces)	246	4	6	32
Milk chocolate and other dark chocolate	235	35	0	16
Cookies, Cakes and Pies, made with white flour and white sugar	varies	varies	0	4 (3) – 8 (5)

FAST FOODS AND SNACKS

	CALORIES	SODIUM (mg)	NUT. IQ	ANDI
Popcorn (4 cups)	257	466	0	14
Potato chips (1 ounce)	154	136	0	13
Pretzels (1 ounce)	108	385	0	12 (5)
Corn chips (1 ounce)	147	155	0	7
Chicken or beef burritos (1 item)	490	1250	0	19
Cheese Pizza (2 slices)	483	1354	0	15 (12)
Fast Food Hamburger (1 item)	265	532	0	12 (9)
Fast Food Cheeseburger (1 item)	313	745	0	12 (9)
Fast food chicken sandwich (1 item)	524	1178	0	12 (11)
Chicken or beef tacos (2 tacos)	340	620	0	12
Bacon, Egg and Cheese Biscuit (1 item)	432	1225	0	11 (9)
Fast food fish sandwich (1 item)	391	689	0	8 (6)
French fries (1 medium serving)	370	266	0	9
Milk shake (12 fl oz)	419	142	0	10

	CALORIES	SODIUM (mg)	NUT. IQ	ANDI

BEVERAGES

	CALORIES	SODIUM (mg)	NUT. IQ	ANDI
Red wine (4 ounces)	100	5	0	30
White wine (4 ounces)	96	6	0	7
Beer (12 ounces)	153	14	0	7
Cola (8 ounces)	91	10	0	1

SPREADS

	CALORIES	SODIUM (mg)	NUT. IQ	ANDI
Jam/preserves (1 tablespoon)	56	6	0	4
Butter (1 tablespoon)	102	101	0	3
Jelly (1 tablespoon)	56	6	0	2

SWEETENERS

	CALORIES	SODIUM (mg)	NUT. IQ	ANDI
Maple syrup, (2 tablespoons)	104	5	0	15
Brown sugar (1 tablespoon)	34	3	0	1
Corn syrup (2 tablespoons)	125	27	0	0
White sugar (1 tablespoon)	49	0	0	0

OILS

	CALORIES	SODIUM (mg)	NUT. IQ	ANDI
Olive oil (1 tablespoon)	119	0	0	10
Sunflower oil (1 tablespoon)	120	0	0	8
Corn/Canola oil (1 tablespoon)	124	0	0	2

Note:

In some cases, scores may vary between raw and cooked foods for Nutrient IQ scores but not for ANDI because Nutrient IQ is based on a measured amount. For example, you consume more with one cup of cooked kale than one cup of raw kale.

Many processed foods in the Refined Grains, Breads and Crackers, Cereals, Fast Foods and Snacks categories are enriched or fortified with B-complex vitamins, iron and other nutrients. Enrichment and fortification put back only a small percentage of the hundreds of valuable health-promoting components lost during processing. Processing and refining also create unhealthy compounds not found in whole, natural foods. In my ANDI scores for processed, refined foods, I have included estimates in parenthesis of what the ANDI would be without artificial enrichment or fortification. This gives you a more accurate picture of the insignificant nutritional value of these foods.

Chapter Seven

NUTRIENT-RICH MENUS

Earlier, we discussed my two levels of nutritional excellence. In this chapter, we will do a sample menu comparison of Nutritarian against standard American diet for the two levels. Portions should be adjusted according to caloric needs.

All recipes with an asterisk are available in Chapter Eight, High Nutrient Recipes, beginning on Page 79.

LEVEL ONE
GOOD

Standard American Diet	**Nutritarian Diet**

BREAKFAST

    Blueberry muffin

    Coffee with cream

LUNCH

    Cheeseburger on a bun

    French fries

    Iced tea

DINNER

    Fried chicken

    Cole slaw

    Corn

    Roll

    Cookies

BREAKFAST

    Blueberry Banana
    Breakfast Cobbler*

LUNCH

    Teff Burgers* on a
    whole grain bun

    Shredded Cabbage
    Slaw*

    Watermelon

DINNER

    Big Salad (romaine,
    arugula, tomato and
    red onion) with
    Almond Vinaigrette
    Dressing*

    Black Bean Quinoa
    Soup*

    Steamed broccoli

    Nutritarian Chocolate
    Chip Cookies*

NUTRITIONAL ANALYSIS

	SAD	Nutritarian
Nutrient IQ Score	139	778
Calories	2335	2054
Protein (g)	87	84
Carbohydrate (g)	276	333
Fat (g)	102	59
Cholesterol (mg)	257	0
Saturated fat (g)	26	10
Fiber (g)	19	67
Sodium (mg)	2627	1044
Vitamin C (mg)	31	268
B1, thiamine (mg)	1.5	4.6
B6, pyridoxine (mg)	1.5	2.7
Iron (mg)	14	26
Folate (mg)	348	900
Magnesium (mg)	186	798
Calcium (mg)	515	683
Zinc (mg)	9	14
Selenium (mcg)	117	91
Alpha tocopherol (mcg)	4.5	18
Beta carotene (mcg)	82	14841
Alpha Carotene (mcg)	28	1793
Lutein & Zeaxanthin (mcg)	1174	15575
Lycopene (mcg)	0	14433

LEVEL TWO
GREAT

Standard American Diet	**Nutritarian Diet**

BREAKFAST

Bagel with cream cheese

Caramel Latte

LUNCH

Cobb Salad (with lettuce, tomato, bacon, avocado, chicken, hard-boiled egg and blue cheese)

Diet soda

DINNER

Rib eye steak

Baked potato with sour cream

Green beans

Apple pie with vanilla ice cream

BREAKFAST

Super Green Smoothie*

Mixed fruit cup topped with walnuts

LUNCH

Big Salad (mixed greens, shredded cabbage, tomato and red onion) and Creamy Avocado Dressing*

Two Bean Chili*

Sliced mango

DINNER

Mushroom and White Bean Loaf*

Cauliflower Spinach Mashed "Potatoes"*

Kale sautéed with garlic

Chia Pudding with fresh raspberries*

NUTRITIONAL ANALYSIS

	SAD	Nutritarian
Nutrient IQ Score	208	1294
Calories	3003	2117
Protein (g)	105	79
Carbohydrate (g)	248	313
Fat (g)	180	82
Cholesterol (mg)	680	0
Saturated fat (g)	74	16
Fiber (g)	18	87
Sodium (mg)	2327	578
Vitamin C (mg)	48	720
B1, thiamine (mg)	1.3	3.4
B6, pyridoxine (mg)	2.2	4.0
Iron (mg)	16	30
Folate (mg)	545	1238
Magnesium (mg)	226	970
Calcium (mg)	1079	1377
Zinc (mg)	13	15
Selenium (mcg)	113	54
Alpha tocopherol (mcg)	8.5	11.7
Beta carotene (mcg)	4622	47,674
Alpha Carotene (mcg)	70	7040
Lutein & Zeaxanthin (mcg)	3098	68,347
Lycopene (mcg)	1312	7202

Chapter Eight

NUTRIENT-RICH RECIPES

My high-nutrient recipes are among the most healthful in the world. And they taste great! The recipes that follow are just a sampling to get you started. You can find many more delicious recipes on my website, DrFuhrman.com. As a member of DrFuhrman.com, you'll have access to targeted meal plans and more than 2,000 recipes, which are rated and commented on by other members.

Feel free to adjust or add herbs and spices to suit your tastes – just don't add salt. Nutrient IQ points are given in convenient kitchen measures and are not necessarily recommended serving amounts. Adjust the scores based the size of your serving.

SMOOTHIES AND JUICES

BLUEBERRY ORANGE SMOOTHIE   *Serves 1*

1 orange, peeled and seeded

1/2 banana (frozen or fresh)

1/2 cup frozen blueberries

1 tablespoon ground flax seeds

2 cups chopped kale or baby bok choy

Blend all ingredients together in a high-powered blender until smooth and creamy.

NUTRIENT IQ POINTS: 137 per cup

CALORIES 265; PROTEIN 8g; CARBOHYDRATES 56g; SUGARS 26g; TOTAL FAT 4.8g; SATURATED FAT 0.5g; SODIUM 62mg; FIBER 11.3g; BETA-CAROTENE 12522ug; VITAMIN C 251mg; CALCIUM 268mg; IRON 3.2mg; FOLATE 110ug; MAGNESIUM 108mg; POTASSIUM 1141mg; ZINC 1.1mg; SELENIUM 3.7ug

CHOCOLATE PEANUT BUTTER SMOOTHIE   *Serves: 1*

2 cups chopped kale
1 tablespoon no-salt-added peanut butter
1 tablespoon unsweetened cocoa powder
1/2 ripe frozen banana
1/2-1 cup unsweetened soy, hemp or almond milk*
1/4 teaspoon pure vanilla bean powder

Blend all ingredients in high-powered blender.

*Adjust the amount of non-dairy milk to desired consistency. For added sweetness, add 1-2 pitted dates.

NUTRIENT IQ POINTS: 75 per cup

CALORIES 269; PROTEIN 14g; CARBOHYDRATES 35g; SUGARS 9g; TOTAL FAT 11.9g; SATURATED FAT 2.5g; SODIUM 107mg; FIBER 7.6g; BETA-CAROTENE 12378ug; VITAMIN C 166mg; CALCIUM 351mg; IRON 4mg; FOLATE 64ug; MAGNESIUM 133mg; POTASSIUM 1145mg; ZINC 2mg; SELENIUM 3.5ug

(Unsweetened almond milk used for calculations.)

Super Green Smoothie   *Serves: 1*

>   2 cups chopped green cruciferous vegetable (kale,
>   collards, mustard greens or turnip greens)
>   1/3 cup broccoli or radish sprouts*
>   6 walnut halves
>   1 1/2 tablespoons hemp seeds
>   1 cup frozen strawberries, raspberries or other berries
>   1 cup carrot or beet juice*
>   squeeze of lemon

Blend ingredients in a high-powered blender until
smooth.

*If you don't have sprouts you can leave them out; if you
don't have beet or carrot juice, you can substitute half a
cup (each) of pomegranate juice and unsweetened soy,
hemp or almond milk – or just one cup of the non-dairy
milk.

NUTRIENT IQ POINTS: 157 per cup

CALORIES 337; PROTEIN 12g; CARBOHYDRATES 52g; SUGARS 18g; TOTAL FAT
13g; SATURATED FAT 1.3g; SODIUM 176mg; FIBER 13.4g; BETA-CAROTENE
24961ug; VITAMIN C 288mg; CALCIUM 297mg; IRON 5.7mg; FOLATE 145ug;
MAGNESIUM 180mg; POTASSIUM 1666mg; ZINC 2.7mg; SELENIUM 4.2ug

GO-TO GREEN JUICE   *Serves: 2*

2 cucumbers

2 large carrots

10 organic kale leaves

1 green apple, cored and cut in quarters

1 lemon, peeled

Wash all ingredients. Run all ingredients through a juicer.

NUTRIENT IQ POINTS: 116 per cup

CALORIES 152; PROTEIN 8g; CARBOHYDRATES 33g; SUGARS 16g; TOTAL FAT 1.9g; SATURATED FAT 0.2g; SODIUM 112mg; BETA-CAROTENE 19694ug; VITAMIN C 228mg; CALCIUM 283mg; IRON 3.7mg; FOLATE 100ug; MAGNESIUM 98mg; POTASSIUM 1360mg; ZINC 1.3mg; SELENIUM 1.8ug

BREAKFASTS

APPLE PIE OATMEAL   *Serves 1*

1 apple, peeled, cored, and diced

1 cup water (for old fashioned oats) or 2 cups water (for steel cut oats)

1/2 cup old fashioned or steel cut oats

1/4 teaspoon ground cinnamon

2 tablespoons chopped walnuts

1/4 teaspoon pure vanilla bean powder

Place apples and water in a small pot over medium heat. Add oats just before it reaches a gentle boil. Reduce heat to low and simmer for 5 minutes for old fashioned oats and 20 minutes for steel cut oats, stirring occasionally.

Add more water if needed to adjust consistency to your liking. Remove from heat and stir in cinnamon, walnuts and vanilla.

NUTRIENT IQ POINTS: 46 per cup

CALORIES 281 PROTEIN 7G CARBOHYDRATES 49G SUGARS 16G TOTAL FAT 8.5G SATURATED FAT 1G CHOLESTEROL 0MG SODIUM 10MG FIBER 6.9G BETA-CAROTENE 29UG VITAMIN C 7MG CALCIUM 29MG IRON 10.6MG FOLATE 8UG MAGNESIUM 22MG POTASSIUM 183MG ZINC 0.5MG SELENIUM 0.4UG

BLUEBERRY BANANA BREAKFAST COBBLER *Serves 2*

> 1 banana, sliced
> 1 cup frozen blueberries
> 1/4 cup old fashioned rolled oats
> 1 tablespoon dried currants
> 1/8 teaspoon pure vanilla bean powder
> 2 tablespoons chopped raw almonds
> 2 tablespoons unsweetened, shredded coconut
> 1/4 teaspoon cinnamon

Combine banana, berries, oats, currants and vanilla in a microwave-safe dish. Microwave for 2 minutes. Top with almonds, coconut and cinnamon and microwave for 1 minute. Serve warm.

NUTRIENT IQ POINTS: 65 per cup

CALORIES 216; PROTEIN 4g; CARBOHYDRATES 36g; SUGARS 17g; TOTAL FAT 8.1g; SATURATED FAT 3.7g; SODIUM 4mg; FIBER 6.8g; BETA-CAROTENE 39ug; VITAMIN C 7mg; CALCIUM 34mg; IRON 3.4mg; FOLATE 21ug; MAGNESIUM 43mg; POTASSIUM 368mg; ZINC 0.5mg; SELENIUM 1.9ug

QUICK BREAKFAST QUINOA BOWL   *Serves 4*

1 cup dry quinoa

2 cups water

1 medium apple, cored and diced

1/2 cup raw almonds, chopped

1 cup fresh or thawed frozen blueberries

1/2 cup raisins or chopped, pitted dates

1 teaspoon cinnamon

1/2 cup unsweetened soy, hemp or almond milk

Place quinoa and water in a saucepan, bring to a boil, cover, reduce heat, and simmer for 15 minutes or until quinoa is tender and all the water is absorbed. Fluff with a fork.

Add remaining ingredients and cook for another 2-3 minutes, stirring frequently. Divide among four bowls.

NUTRIENT IQ POINTS: 46 per cup

CALORIES 332; PROTEIN 10g; CARBOHYDRATES 57g; SUGARS 20g; TOTAL FAT 9.1g; SATURATED FAT 0.8g; SODIUM 33mg; FIBER 7.8g; BETA-CAROTENE 30ug; VITAMIN C 4mg; CALCIUM 140mg; IRON 3mg; FOLATE 90ug; MAGNESIUM 129mg; POTASSIUM 539mg; ZINC 1.8mg; SELENIUM 4.1ug

(Unsweetened almond milk used for calculations.)

SCRAMBLED TOFU WITH RED PEPPER, TOMATO AND SPINACH

Serves 2

3 scallions, diced

1/2 cup finely chopped red bell pepper

1 medium tomato, chopped

2 cloves garlic, minced or pressed

14 ounces firm tofu, drained and crumbled

1 tablespoon *Dr. Fuhrman's MatoZest* or other no-salt seasoning blend, adjusted to taste

1 tablespoon nutritional yeast

5 ounces baby spinach, coarsely chopped

1 teaspoon coconut aminos

In a large skillet, over medium/high heat, sauté scallions, red pepper, tomato, and garlic in 1/4 cup water for 5 minutes. Add remaining ingredients and cook for another 5 minutes.

If desired, serve with *Dr. Fuhrman's no-salt, no-sugar Ketchup.*

NUTRIENT IQ POINTS: 102 per cup

CALORIES 249; PROTEIN 24g; CARBOHYDRATES 19g; SUGARS 6g; TOTAL FAT 9.7g; SATURATED FAT 1.1g; SODIUM 148mg; FIBER 6.7g; BETA-CAROTENE 5003ug; VITAMIN C 84mg; CALCIUM 367mg; IRON 5.7mg; FOLATE 194ug; MAGNESIUM 86mg; POTASSIUM 694mg; ZINC 1.6mg; SELENIUM 1.6ug

SOUPS AND STEWS

BLACK BEAN QUINOA SOUP   *Serves 4*

1 medium onion, chopped

1 green bell pepper, chopped

1 large carrot, chopped

4 cloves garlic, minced

1 cup chopped fresh tomato

1 teaspoon ground cumin

2 teaspoons chili powder

1/4 teaspoon crushed red pepper flakes

5 cups low-sodium or no-salt-added vegetable broth

1/2 cup quinoa, rinsed

3 cups cooked black beans or 2 (15 ounce) cans no-salt-added black beans, drained

4 cups spinach or thinly sliced kale

1/4 cup chopped cilantro

1 tablespoon fresh lime juice

1 avocado, chopped

In a soup pot, combine onion, green pepper, carrots, garlic, tomatoes, cumin, chili powder, red pepper flakes and vegetable broth. Bring to a boil, reduce heat and cook for 5 minutes. Stir in quinoa, cover and cook for 10 minutes. Add black beans and continue cooking until heated through and quinoa is tender, about 10 minutes. Add spinach or kale and stir until wilted.

Remove from heat and stir in cilantro and lime juice. Serve garnished with chopped avocado.

NUTRIENT IQ POINTS: 79 per cup

CALORIES 372; PROTEIN 19g; CARBOHYDRATES 65g; SUGARS 4g; TOTAL FAT 5.6g; SATURATED FAT 0.8g; SODIUM 244mg; FIBER 17.9g; BETA-CAROTENE 8221ug; VITAMIN C 118mg; CALCIUM 203mg; IRON 6.4mg; FOLATE 286ug; MAGNESIUM 178mg; POTASSIUM 1279mg; ZINC 2.8mg; SELENIUM 4.9ug

CREAMY MUSHROOM SOUP   *Serves 4*

20 ounces white or brown mushrooms, sliced

1 cup carrot juice

2 cups no-salt-added or low-sodium vegetable broth

1 large sweet onion

2 small carrots, sliced

2 tablespoons *Dr.Fuhrman's Vegizest* or other no-salt seasoning blend, adjusted to taste

1 1/2 teaspoons coconut aminos

4 cloves garlic, pressed

2 tablespoons fresh cilantro

1 cup walnuts

2 cups unsweetened soy, hemp or almond milk

1/4 teaspoon black pepper, or to taste

Combine all ingredients except cilantro, walnuts, non-dairy milk and black pepper in a large pot. Cook about 25 minutes or until carrots and mushrooms are tender. Remove from heat and stir in fresh cilantro.

Pour 3/4 of the soup in a high-powered blender with the walnuts and non-dairy milk. Blend until smooth. Pour mixture back into pot, stir and heat through. Season with black pepper.

NUTRIENT IQ POINTS: 79 per cup

CALORIES 331; PROTEIN 12g; CARBOHYDRATES 30g; SUGARS 12g; TOTAL FAT 21.2g; SATURATED FAT 1.9g; SODIUM 291mg; FIBER 6g; BETA-CAROTENE 7585ug; VITAMIN C 18mg; CALCIUM 347mg; IRON 3.3mg; FOLATE 77ug; MAGNESIUM 97mg; POTASSIUM 1035mg; ZINC 2.1mg; SELENIUM 16.1ug

LEMON LENTIL SOUP
Serves 4

1 1/2 cups carrots, peeled and chopped

1 cup celery, chopped

4 cups no-salt-added or low-sodium vegetable broth

1 cup red lentils, rinsed and drained

3/4 teaspoon ground coriander

1 teaspoon ground cumin

3 tablespoons raw cashews

1/4 cup fresh lemon juice (about 2 small lemons)

1 head baby bok choy, chopped (could substitute
2 cups chopped greens, such as kale or spinach)

2 tablespoons chopped parsley

black pepper, to taste

Place carrots, celery, vegetable broth, lentils, coriander and cumin in a pot and bring to a boil. Reduce heat, cover and simmer for 40 minutes or until lentils and vegetables are tender.

In a blender or food processor, blend 1 cup of the soup with cashews and lemon juice. Return to pot along with bok choy or greens and heat until greens are wilted. Stir in parsley and season with pepper.

NUTRIENT IQ POINTS: 58 per cup

CALORIES 301; PROTEIN 22g; CARBOHYDRATES 45g; SUGARS 7g; TOTAL FAT 5.5g; SATURATED FAT 1.1g; SODIUM 268mg; FIBER 19g; BETA-CAROTENE 9787ug; VITAMIN C 109mg; CALCIUM 296mg; IRON 7mg; FOLATE 394ug; MAGNESIUM

TOMATO FLORENTINE SOUP   *Serves 4*

1 large onion, chopped

1 celery stalk, chopped

3 garlic cloves, minced

5 cups low-sodium or no-salt-added vegetable broth

3 cups diced fresh tomatoes, undrained or 1 (26 ounce) carton diced tomatoes (see note)

6 ounces (3/4 cup) tomato paste (see note)

3 tablespoons raisins, minced

1 1/2 cups cooked great northern beans or 1 (15 ounce) can no-salt-added great northern beans, drained

5 ounces spinach

5 ounces baby kale

1/4 teaspoon ground black pepper, or to taste

1/4 cup nutritional yeast

6 medium fresh basil leaves, finely chopped

In a soup pot, combine onion, celery, garlic, broth, tomatoes, tomato paste, and raisins. Bring to a boil, reduce heat and simmer for about 20 minutes, stirring occasionally.

Add beans, spinach, kale, pepper, nutritional yeast, and basil. Stir to combine. Simmer until greens are wilted and soup is heated through. Additional vegetable broth can be added to adjust consistency.

Note: Select tomatoes packed in glass or cartons. These materials do not contain BPA.

NUTRIENT IQ POINTS: 88 per cup

CALORIES 248; PROTEIN 15g; CARBOHYDRATES 46g; SUGARS 15g; TOTAL FAT 1.6g; SATURATED FAT 0.3g; SODIUM 227mg; FIBER 12.2g; BETA-CAROTENE 6304ug; VITAMIN C 85mg; CALCIUM 208mg; IRON 5.7mg; FOLATE 184ug; MAGNESIUM 125mg; POTASSIUM 1511mg; ZINC 3.1mg; SELENIUM 6.3ug

TWO BEAN CHILI   *Serves 4*

1 cup chopped onion

1/2 cup chopped green bell pepper, fresh or frozen

1 clove garlic, chopped

3/4 cup water

2 tablespoons tomato paste

1 tablespoon chili powder

2 teaspoons ground cumin

1/4 teaspoon black pepper

1 1/2 cups cooked or 1 (15 ounce) can no-salt-added black beans, drained

3 cups cooked or 2 (15 ounce) cans no-salt-added red pinto or kidney beans, drained

2 cups no-salt-added vegetable broth

1 1/2 cups diced tomatoes

1 tablespoon yellow cornmeal

Water sauté onion and bell pepper in a soup pot until almost tender. Add garlic and cook for another minute. Stir in water, tomato paste, chili powder, cumin, black pepper, beans, vegetable broth and diced tomatoes and bring to a boil. Reduce heat, cover and simmer for 10 minutes. Stir in cornmeal and cook for an additional two minutes.

Note: If desired, 1 cup of frozen corn and/or frozen chopped broccoli may be added before soup is simmered.

NUTRIENT IQ POINTS: 88 per cup

CALORIES 317; PROTEIN 19g; CARBOHYDRATES 59g; SUGARS 6g; TOTAL FAT 1.9g; SATURATED FAT 0.3g; SODIUM 119mg; FIBER 18.6g; BETA-CAROTENE 725ug; VITAMIN C 31mg; CALCIUM 107mg; IRON 7.2mg; FOLATE 290ug; MAGNESIUM 132mg; POTASSIUM 1164mg; ZINC 2.6mg; SELENIUM 3.9ug

SALAD DRESSINGS AND SAUCES

<u>CREAMY AVOCADO DRESSING</u> *Serves 4*

> 2 ripe avocados, peeled, pitted and chopped
> 2 tablespoons nutritional yeast
> 1/4 cup unsweetened soy, hemp or almond milk
> 2-3 small shallots, according to taste
> 1/4 cup white wine vinegar

Blend all ingredients in a high-powered blender until smooth and creamy.

You can modify amounts of shallot and non-dairy milk to adjust taste and consistency.

NUTRIENT IQ POINTS: 9 per tablespoon

CALORIES 143; PROTEIN 4g; CARBOHYDRATES 9g; SUGARS 1g; TOTAL FAT 10.9g; SATURATED FAT 1.5g; SODIUM 14mg; FIBER 5.8g; BETA-CAROTENE 43ug; VITAMIN C 7mg; CALCIUM 35mg; IRON 0.8mg; FOLATE 64ug; MAGNESIUM 30mg; POTASSIUM 397mg; ZINC 1.4mg; SELENIUM 0.5ug

(Unsweetened almond milk used for calculations.)

ALMOND VINAIGRETTE DRESSING   *Serves 6*

    1 cup unsweetened soy, hemp or almond milk
    3/4 cup raw almonds
    2 tablespoons hemp seeds
    1/4 cup balsamic vinegar
    2 tablespoons fresh lemon juice
    1/4 cup raisins
    2 teaspoons Dijon mustard
    1 clove garlic

Blend ingredients in a high-powered blender until creamy and smooth.

NUTRIENT IQ POINTS: 4 per tablespoon

CALORIES 181; PROTEIN 7g; CARBOHYDRATES 13g; SUGARS 6g; TOTAL FAT 12.5g; SATURATED FAT 1g; SODIUM 38mg; FIBER 3.4g; BETA-CAROTENE 1ug; VITAMIN C 2mg; CALCIUM 122mg; IRON 1.3mg; FOLATE 13ug; MAGNESIUM 75mg; POTASSIUM 284mg; ZINC 0.9mg; SELENIUM 1.3ug

(Unsweetened almond milk used for calculations.)

ORANGE SESAME DRESSING   *Serves 4*

> 4 tablespoons unhulled sesame seeds, divided
> 2 navel oranges, peeled
> 1/4 cup *Dr. Fuhrman's Blood Orange Vinegar* or white wine vinegar
> 1/4 cup raw cashews
> 1 tablespoon lemon juice, optional

Lightly toast the sesame seeds in a dry skillet over medium high heat for about 3 minutes, shaking the pan frequently.

In a high-powered blender, combine oranges, vinegar, cashews, lemon juice (if desired) and 2 tablespoons of the sesame seeds.

Toss with the salad, sprinkling remaining sesame seeds on top.

Serving Suggestion: Toss with mixed greens, shredded cabbage, tomatoes, red onions and additional diced oranges or kiwi.

NUTRIENT IQ POINTS: 4 per tablespoon

CALORIES 137; PROTEIN 4g; CARBOHYDRATES 14g; SUGARS 7g; TOTAL FAT 8.3g; SATURATED FAT 1.3g; SODIUM 3mg; FIBER 2.9g; BETA-CAROTENE 61ug; VITAMIN C 43mg; CALCIUM 122mg; IRON 2mg; FOLATE 35ug; MAGNESIUM 65mg; POTASSIUM 229mg; ZINC 1.3mg; SELENIUM 4.8ug

BEET HUMMUS   *Serves 6*

1 small beet, peeled and diced
2 cups cooked or no-salt-added canned chickpeas
3 tablespoons tahini or unhulled sesame seeds
1/2 cup water
1 lemon, juiced and zested
2 cloves garlic, chopped
1/2 teaspoon black pepper
chopped dill for garnish
sesame seeds for garnish

In a small pot, bring water to a boil, add diced beets and cook until tender, about 10 minutes. Drain and cool completely.

Place cooked beets in a food processor or blender along with chickpeas, tahini, water, lemon juice, lemon zest, garlic and black pepper and pulse until pureed completely. Add additional water if needed to adjust consistency.

Transfer to a serving dish and refrigerate for 1-2 hours. Garnish with fresh chopped dill and sesame seeds.

NUTRIENT IQ POINTS: 33 per ¼ cup

CALORIES 142; PROTEIN 6g; CARBOHYDRATES 19g; SUGARS 4g; TOTAL FAT 5.4g; SATURATED FAT 0.7g; SODIUM 16mg; FIBER 5.3g; BETA-CAROTENE 15ug; VITAMIN C 6mg; CALCIUM 43mg; IRON 2.2mg; FOLATE 118ug; MAGNESIUM 55mg; POTASSIUM 253mg; ZINC 1.6mg; SELENIUM 2.3ug

CASHEW ALFREDO SAUCE · *Serves 4*

1 cup raw cashews

2 tablespoons unhulled sesame seeds

1 1/2 cups unsweetened soy, hemp or almond milk

3 tablespoons *Dr. Fuhrman's Unfortified Nutritional Yeast* (or other nutritional yeast)

2 tablespoons lemon juice or more to taste

1 teaspoon *Dr. Fuhrman's VegiZest* or other no-salt seasoning blend, adjusted to taste

1 tablespoon chopped garlic or to taste

Blend all ingredients in a high-powered blender. Add more non-dairy milk if needed to adjust consistency. It should be fairly thick but still pour out of the blender.

Serve over steamed vegetables, bean pasta or salads.

NUTRIENT IQ POINTS: 4 per tablespoon

CALORIES 258; PROTEIN 11g; CARBOHYDRATES 15g; SUGARS 2g; TOTAL FAT 18.5g; SATURATED FAT 3g; SODIUM 78mg; FIBER 3g; VITAMIN C 4mg; CALCIUM 261mg; IRON 3.6mg; FOLATE 18ug; MAGNESIUM 132mg; POTASSIUM 262mg; ZINC 3.6mg; SELENIUM 8.7ug

(Unsweetened almond milk used for calculations.)

SALADS

Farro, Mushroom and Arugula Salad *Serves 4*

- 1 cup uncooked farro
- 10 ounces mushrooms, sliced
- 1/4 cup chopped red onion
- 3 cups baby arugula

For the Dressing:
- 1 medium tomato
- 1/3 cup raw cashews
- 1 tablespoon hemp seeds
- 1/4 cup water
- 1/2 lime, juiced
- 1 tablespoon balsamic vinegar

In a saucepan, heat 2 cups of water to boiling. Stir in farro; return to a boil. Reduce heat to low, cover and cook for 20 to 25 minutes or until farro is tender. Drain. Meanwhile, water sauté the mushrooms until they are soft and lightly browned. Combine cooked farro, mushrooms, chopped onion and arugula. Blend dressing ingredients together in a high-powered blender. Add desired amount of dressing to salad and toss. Serve warm or at room temperature.

NUTRIENT IQ POINTS: 118 per cup

CALORIES 311; PROTEIN 13g; CARBOHYDRATES 47g; SUGARS 4g; TOTAL FAT 8.1g; SATURATED FAT 1.1g; SODIUM 13mg; FIBER 9.2g; BETA-CAROTENE 354ug; VITAMIN C 11mg; CALCIUM 61mg; IRON 3.5mg; FOLATE 39ug; MAGNESIUM 69mg; POTASSIUM 485mg; ZINC 1.4mg; SELENIUM 9ug

Kale and Red Cabbage Salad with Apples and Dried Cherries

Serves 2

- 1 bunch kale, tough stems and center ribs removed
- 1 avocado, peeled and chopped
- 2 tablespoons lemon juice
- 1 tablespoon white balsamic vinegar
- 1 cup thinly sliced red cabbage
- 1 large apple, cored and chopped
- 2 tablespoons chopped unsweetened dried cherries or raisins
- 1/2 medium red onion, minced
- 2 tablespoons chives, chopped

Roll up each kale leaf and slice thinly. Add to bowl along with avocado, lemon juice and vinegar. Using your hands, massage the avocado, lemon juice and vinegar into the kale leaves until the kale starts to soften and wilt and each leaf is coated, about 2 to 3 minutes.

Mix in red cabbage, apple, dried cherries, onion and chives.

NUTRIENT IQ POINTS: 156 per cup

CALORIES 317; PROTEIN 8g; CARBOHYDRATES 53g; SUGARS 16g; TOTAL FAT 12g; SATURATED FAT 1.7g; SODIUM 92mg; FIBER 12.4g; BETA-CAROTENE 15840ug; VITAMIN C 244mg; CALCIUM 270mg; IRON 3.9mg; FOLATE 130ug; MAGNESIUM 94mg; POTASSIUM 1372mg; ZINC 1.4mg; SELENIUM 2.2ug

Shredded Cabbage Slaw   *Serves 4*

1/4 small red cabbage, thinly shredded
1/2 small green cabbage, thinly shredded
1 carrot, shredded
1/4 cup finely chopped onion
1 teaspoon celery seed

For the Dressing

1/2 cup raw cashews
2 tablespoons hemp seeds
1/4 cup raisins or currants
1/2 cup unsweetened soy, hemp or almond milk
2 cloves garlic
2 tablespoons apple cider vinegar
2 tablespoons lemon juice
1 teaspoon Dijon mustard

In a large bowl, mix together red and green cabbage, carrot, onion and celery seed.

Blend remaining ingredients in a high-powered blender. Toss cabbage mixture with desired amount of dressing.

NUTRIENT IQ POINTS: 110 per cup

CALORIES 151; PROTEIN 5g; CARBOHYDRATES 20g; SUGARS 10g; TOTAL FAT 6.7g; SATURATED FAT 1.2g; SODIUM 57mg; FIBER 3.8g; BETA-CAROTENE 1232ug; VITAMIN C 46mg; CALCIUM 72mg; IRON 2mg; FOLATE 49ug; MAGNESIUM 67mg; POTASSIUM 433mg; ZINC 1.1mg; SELENIUM 4.9ug

(Unsweetened almond milk used for calculations.)

THREE BEAN MANGO SALAD   *Serves 6*

1 1/2 cups cooked or 1 (15 ounce) can no-salt-added cannellini beans, drained

1 1/2 cups cooked or 1 (15 ounce) can no-salt-added kidney beans, drained

1 1/2 cups cooked or 1 (15 ounce) can no-salt-added chickpeas, drained

2 mangoes, peeled, pitted and cubed

1/2 red onion, finely chopped

1/2 red bell pepper, chopped

1/2 cup finely chopped flat leaf parsley

10 ounces mixed baby greens

For the Dressing

1/2 cup water

1/3 cup cider vinegar

1/4 cup raw almonds

1/4 cup raisins

2 teaspoons whole grain mustard

1/2 teaspoon dried oregano

In a large bowl, mix the beans, mangoes, onion, bell pepper and parsley.

Blend water, vinegar, almonds, raisins, mustard and oregano in a high-powered blender until smooth. Add dressing to bean mixture and toss to coat.

Chill in the refrigerator for several hours, to allow beans to soak up the flavor of the dressing.

Serve on top of the mixed greens.

NUTRIENT IQ POINTS: 86 per cup

CALORIES 328; PROTEIN 16g; CARBOHYDRATES 59g; SUGARS 23g; TOTAL FAT 5.1g; SATURATED FAT 0.6g; SODIUM 50mg; FIBER 12.5g; BETA-CAROTENE 3912ug; VITAMIN C 69mg; CALCIUM 153mg; IRON 5.7mg; FOLATE 280ug; MAGNESIUM 119mg; POTASSIUM 1065mg; ZINC 2.4mg; SELENIUM 4.4ug

MAIN DISHES

| Broccoli and Shiitake Mushrooms with Thai Peanut Sauce | *Serves 4* |

For the Thai Peanut Sauce (see note):

1 1/2 cups water

7 regular or 3 1/2 Medjool dates, pitted

1/3 cup no-salt-added peanut butter

2 tablespoons unsweetened shredded coconut

1 teaspoon minced ginger

1 tablespoon lime juice

1 teaspoon red curry powder

1/2 teaspoon chili powder

1/2 teaspoon ground cumin

1/4 teaspoon ground turmeric

For the Vegetables:

1 cup chopped onions

6 cups broccoli florets

1 cup thinly sliced red bell pepper strips

2 cups trimmed snow peas

2 cups sliced shiitake mushrooms

To make the sauce:

Blend water and dates in a high-powered blender, then add peanut butter, coconut, ginger, lime juice and spices and blend again until smooth and well-combined.

To cook the vegetables:

Heat 1/4 cup water in a large non-stick wok or skillet, then add chopped onions and broccoli, cover and cook for 4 minutes, stirring occasionally and adding additional water as needed to prevent sticking. Remove cover and add red bell pepper strips, shiitake mushrooms and snow peas and cook for an additional 4 minutes or until vegetables are crisp-tender. Add desired amount of sauce and continue to stir fry for 1-2 minutes to heat through.

Note: In a rush? Dr. Fuhrman's time-saving bottled sauces are available at www.drfuhrman.com. *Dr. Fuhrman's Thai Curry Sauce* would work well in this recipe.

NUTRIENT IQ POINTS: 78 per cup

CALORIES 295; PROTEIN 13g; CARBOHYDRATES 39g; SUGARS 18g; TOTAL FAT 13.5g; SATURATED FAT 3.2g; SODIUM 70mg; FIBER 11.4g; BETA-CAROTENE 1123ug; VITAMIN C 174mg; CALCIUM 117mg; IRON 3.4mg; FOLATE 151ug; MAGNESIUM 111mg; POTASSIUM 1152mg; ZINC 2.6mg; SELENIUM 11.9ug

Cauliflower, Spinach Mashed "Potatoes"   *Serves 4*

6 cups fresh or frozen cauliflower florets
2-4 cloves garlic, sliced
10 ounces fresh spinach
1/2 cup raw cashew butter
2 tablespoons hemp seeds
1 teaspoon *Dr. Fuhrman's VegiZest* or other no-salt seasoning blend, adjusted to taste
1/4 teaspoon nutmeg
unsweetened soy, almond or hemp milk, as needed

Steam cauliflower and garlic about 8 to 10 minutes or until tender. Drain and press out as much water as possible in strainer. Place in a high-powered blender or food processor.

Steam spinach until just wilted and set aside.

Blend cauliflower, garlic, cashew butter, hemp seeds, *VegiZest* and nutmeg until smooth and creamy. Add non-dairy milk if needed to adjust consistency. Stir in wilted spinach.

NUTRIENT IQ POINTS: 181 per cup

CALORIES 250; PROTEIN 11g; CARBOHYDRATES 20g; SUGARS 3g; TOTAL FAT 16.6g; SATURATED FAT 3.3g; SODIUM 110mg; FIBER 5.6g; BETA-CAROTENE 3987ug; VITAMIN C 98mg; CALCIUM 125mg; IRON 4.3mg; FOLATE 253ug; MAGNESIUM 165mg; POTASSIUM 1057mg; ZINC 2.5mg; SELENIUM 5.6ug

Collard Greens and Beans — *Serves 2*

1 large onion, sliced
3 cloves garlic, thinly sliced
1 bunch collard greens, stems removed and cut into 1/2 inch strips
1/4 teaspoon red pepper flakes or more to taste
1/2 cup low-sodium or no-salt-added vegetable broth
1 1/2 cups cooked or 1 (15 ounce) can no-salt-added cannellini beans
1 1/2 cups chopped tomato
2 tablespoons lemon juice

Heat 2-3 tablespoons water in a large sauté pan or wok and water sauté onion and garlic until tender. Add collards, red pepper flakes and vegetable broth, cover, and cook for 5 minutes. Add beans, tomatoes and lemon juice, cover and continue cooking for an additional 5 minutes or until collards are wilted and tender. Add additional vegetable broth if needed to prevent sticking.

NUTRIENT IQ POINTS: 166 per cup

CALORIES 276; PROTEIN 17g; CARBOHYDRATES 53g; SUGARS 8g; TOTAL FAT 1.2g; SATURATED FAT 0.2g; SODIUM 67mg; FIBER 14.9g; BETA-CAROTENE 3379ug; VITAMIN C 57mg; CALCIUM 270mg; IRON 5.8mg; FOLATE 264ug; MAGNESIUM 116mg; POTASSIUM 1341mg; ZINC 2.4mg; SELENIUM 3.7ug

Mushroom and White Bean Loaf — *Serves 8*

1 large sweet potato

1 medium onion, finely chopped

2 stalks celery, finely chopped

1 medium carrot, finely chopped

2 cloves garlic, finely chopped

2 cups finely chopped mushrooms

1 1/2 cups cooked or 1 (15 ounce) can no-salt-added cannellini beans, drained

8 ounces extra firm tofu, excess water squeezed out

1/4 cup *Dr. Fuhrman's Ketchup* or other low-sodium ketchup plus additional for top of loaf

1 tablespoon *Dr. Fuhrman's VegiZest* or other no-salt seasoning blend, adjusted to taste

1 tablespoon mustard

1/2 teaspoon poultry seasoning (a blend of sage, thyme, marjoram, rosemary, black pepper and nutmeg)

1/2 teaspoon oregano

1/4 teaspoon black pepper

1 cup old fashioned oats, pulsed in food processor to a coarse powder

1/2 cup chopped pecans

1/4 cup chopped parsley

Pierce sweet potato in several places with a fork and microwave until soft, about 5-6 minutes. When cool enough to handle, peel and set aside.

Heat a large skillet. Add the onion, celery, carrot, garlic and mushrooms and cook, stirring regularly until tender and all the water from the mushrooms has evaporated. Mash beans with a fork and add to the mushroom mixture.

Place the peeled sweet potato into a food processor along with the tofu, ketchup, *VegiZest*, mustard, poultry seasoning, oregano and black pepper. Process until smooth and well combined.

Add tofu mixture to mushrooms and beans along with oats, pecans and parsley and mix well.

Spoon into a loaf pan that has been lightly rubbed with a minimal amount of oil. Spread ketchup on top. Bake at 350 degrees for 1 hour and 10 minutes. Allow to sit for 30 minutes before slicing.

NUTRIENT IQ POINTS: 69 per slice (8 slices/loaf)

CALORIES 217; PROTEIN 11g; CARBOHYDRATES 27g; SUGARS 4g; TOTAL FAT 8.6g; SATURATED FAT 1g; SODIUM 60mg; FIBER 7.6g; BETA-CAROTENE 2201ug; VITAMIN C 7mg; CALCIUM 256mg; IRON 5mg; FOLATE 80ug; MAGNESIUM 63mg; POTASSIUM 519mg; ZINC 1.5mg; SELENIUM 11.4ug

Portobello Pizza   *Serves 1*

2 large Portobello mushrooms, stems removed
1/4 teaspoon garlic powder
1/4 teaspoon dried basil
1/4 teaspoon dried oregano
1/2 cup low-sodium pasta sauce
1/3 cup thinly sliced onion
1/3 cup thinly sliced green or red bell pepper
2-3 tablespoons Nutritarian Parmesan **(see note)**

Preheat oven to 350 degrees F.

Place mushrooms on a parchment-lined baking sheet, gill side up and sprinkle with garlic powder, basil and oregano. Bake for 6 minutes.

Top with tomato sauce, onions and peppers and a sprinkle of Nutritarian Parmesan. Bake for an additional 20 minutes or until vegetables are tender.

Note: To make Nutritarian Parmesan, place 1/4 cup walnuts or almonds and 1/4 cup nutritional yeast in a food processor and pulse until the texture of grated Parmesan is achieved. Store in an airtight container and refrigerate.

NUTRIENT IQ POINTS: 106 per mushroom

CALORIES 179; PROTEIN 11g; CARBOHYDRATES 26g; SUGARS 14g; TOTAL FAT 4.7g; SATURATED FAT 0.6g; CHOLESTEROL 2.6mg; SODIUM 59mg; FIBER 8g; BETA-CAROTENE 569ug; VITAMIN C 30mg; CALCIUM 79mg; IRON 2.6mg; FOLATE 78ug; MAGNESIUM 54mg; POTASSIUM 1178mg; ZINC 3mg; SELENIUM 33.2ug

Spiced Butternut and Brussels Bowl _Serves 4_

    12 ounces butternut squash, cut into 1/2 inch cubes
    1 orange, juiced
    pinch ground cinnamon
    pinch ground cloves
    pinch ground allspice
    pinch cayenne pepper
    1 large shallot, chopped
    3/4 pound Brussel sprouts, shredded or very thinly
    sliced
    1/4 cup toasted pecans, chopped
    2 tablespoons currants or raisins
    2 tablespoons balsamic vinegar
    1/2 teaspoon fresh thyme, chopped
    ground black pepper, to taste

Preheat oven to 350 degrees F.

Mix the squash with the orange juice, cinnamon, cloves, allspice and cayenne. Place the mixture in a baking pan, cover with foil and roast until tender and caramelized but still firm when a fork is inserted, about 20 minutes.

Meanwhile, heat 2 tablespoons water in a large skillet and sauté shallot for 1 minute, add shredded Brussels sprouts and cook for 2-3 minutes, until warm and slightly wilted.

Add a small amount of additional water if needed to prevent from sticking.

Place roasted butternut squash and sautéed Brussels sprouts in a bowl and toss with pecans, currants, vinegar and thyme. Season with black pepper.

NUTRIENT IQ POINTS: 105 per cup

CALORIES 158; PROTEIN 5g; CARBOHYDRATES 28g; SUGARS 11g; TOTAL FAT 4.9g; SATURATED FAT 0.5g; SODIUM 28mg; FIBER 6.2g; BETA-CAROTENE 4006ug; VITAMIN C 106mg; CALCIUM 95mg; IRON 2.3mg; FOLATE 88ug; MAGNESIUM 64mg; POTASSIUM 788mg; ZINC 0.8mg; SELENIUM 2.2ug

Teff Burgers   *Serves 8*

2 cups water
2/3 cup teff **(see note)**
1 cup minced onion
1 cup minced mushrooms
1 medium carrot, grated
1 cup finely chopped kale
1 teaspoon cumin
1 teaspoon chili powder
1/2 teaspoon garlic powder
1/4 teaspoon black pepper
1 1/2 cups cooked or 1 (15 ounce) can no-salt-added red kidney beans, drained
1/4 cup unfortified nutritional yeast

Preheat oven to 350 degrees F.

In a saucepan with a cover, bring water to a boil, stir in teff, reduce to a simmer, cover and cook for 15 minutes or until water is absorbed and teff is tender, stirring occasionally.

In a sauté pan, heat 2 tablespoons of water, add onion and sauté until starting to become translucent, adding more water if needed. Add mushrooms, carrot and kale and cook until mushrooms have released their liquid and the carrots and kale are soft. Stir in cumin, chili powder, garlic powder and black pepper and cook for an additional minute.

Place the beans in a mixing bowl and mash with a fork. Stir in the cooked teff, sautéed vegetables and the nutritional yeast.

Divide the mixture into 8 burgers and place on a parchment or silpat-lined baking pan. Bake for 20 minutes, then turn and bake for an additional 15 minutes.

If desired, serve on a 100% whole grain pita with sliced onion, tomato and lettuce.

Note: Teff is a tiny whole grain with a mild, nutty flavor.

NUTRIENT IQ POINTS: 54 per burger

CALORIES 77; PROTEIN 6g; CARBOHYDRATES 13g; SUGARS 2g; TOTAL FAT 0.6g; SATURATED FAT 0.1g; SODIUM 20mg; FIBER 4.2g; BETA-CAROTENE 1457ug; VITAMIN C 13mg; CALCIUM 36mg; IRON 1.6mg; FOLATE 53ug; MAGNESIUM 29mg; POTASSIUM 267mg; ZINC 1.3mg; SELENIUM 1.5ug

DESSERTS

BANANA MANGO SORBET   *Serves 2*

4 slices unsweetened, unsulfured dried mango (**see note**)
1/4 cup unsweetened soy, hemp or almond milk
1 ripe banana, frozen
2 cups frozen mango
6 ice cubes

Soak dried mango in non-dairy milk until softened, at least one hour.

Add dried mango and soaking liquid to a high-powered blender along with remaining ingredients and blend until creamy but still firm.

If desired, serve topped with walnuts or pecans.

Note: 2 medjool dates or 4 regular dates may be substituted for the dried mango.

NUTRIENT IQ POINTS: 10 per ½ cup

CALORIES 173; PROTEIN 2g; CARBOHYDRATES 43g; SUGARS 33g; TOTAL FAT 1.2g; SATURATED FAT 0.2g; SODIUM 26mg; FIBER 4.2g; BETA-CAROTENE 1223ug; VITAMIN C 65mg; CALCIUM 89mg; IRON 0.7mg; FOLATE 84ug; MAGNESIUM 37mg; POTASSIUM 570mg; ZINC 0.3mg; SELENIUM 1.7ug

(Unsweetened almond milk used for calculations.)

Chia Pudding   *Serves 4*

>1 cup unsweetened soy, hemp or almond milk
>1/2 cup unsweetened, shredded coconut
>1 cup water
>2 medjool or 4 regular dates, pitted
>1/2 teaspoon pure vanilla bean powder
>1/2 - 3/4 teaspoon ground cardamom
>1/2 cup chia seeds, divided

Blend milk, coconut, water, dates, vanilla, cardamom and 1/4 cup of the chia seeds in a high-powered blender. Add additional milk if needed to adjust consistency. Stir in remaining 1/4 cup chia seeds. Refrigerate for 15 minutes and stir again to distribute seeds evenly.

If desired, top with fresh berries and/or toasted unsweetened coconut. For a parfait, alternate layers of berries with pudding in a wine glass. For a chocolate chia pudding, blend in 2 tablespoons natural cocoa powder.

NUTRIENT IQ POINTS: 22 per ½ cup

CALORIES 280; PROTEIN 7g; CARBOHYDRATES 34g; SUGARS 19g; TOTAL FAT 15g; SATURATED FAT 7.3g; SODIUM 42mg; FIBER 11.1g; BETA-CAROTENE 23ug; VITAMIN C 1mg; CALCIUM 171mg; IRON 2.7mg; FOLATE 16ug; MAGNESIUM 111mg; POTASSIUM 391mg; ZINC 1.4mg; SELENIUM 16.8ug

(Unsweetened almond milk used for calculations.)

CHOCOLATE CHERRY ICE CREAM   *Serves 2*

   1/2 cup unsweetened vanilla soy, hemp or almond milk
   1 tablespoon natural, non-alkalized cocoa powder
   4 regular dates or 2 Medjool dates, pitted
   1 1/2 cups frozen dark sweet cherries
   1/2 tablespoon pure vanilla bean powder

Blend all ingredients together in a high-powered blender
or food processor until smooth and creamy.

NUTRIENT IQ POINTS: 26 per ½ cup

CALORIES 120; PROTEIN 4g; CARBOHYDRATES 26g; SUGARS 20g; TOTAL FAT
1.9g; SATURATED FAT 0.5g; SODIUM 25mg; FIBER 4.2g; BETA-CAROTENE 608ug;
VITAMIN C 2mg; CALCIUM 101mg; IRON 1.4mg; FOLATE 9ug; MAGNESIUM 40mg;
POTASSIUM 352mg; ZINC 0.6mg; SELENIUM 0.8ug

(Unsweetened almond milk used for calculations.)

NUTRITARIAN CHOCOLATE CHIP COOKIES   *Serves 10*

1 1/2 cups cooked or 1 (15 ounce) can no- salt- added chickpeas, drained
1/2 cup raw almonds
3/4 cup dates
1 apple, cored
1 teaspoon pure vanilla bean powder
1/4 cup water
2/3 cup old fashioned rolled oats
2/3 cup 100% cacao chocolate chips

Preheat oven to 350 degrees F.

Blend chickpeas, almonds, dates, apple, vanilla and water in a high-powered blender until smooth.

Place in a bowl and mix in oats and chocolate chips.

Drop on a lightly-oiled or parchment-lined baking sheet in 2 tablespoon scoopfuls. Flatten a little with a fork.

Bake for 10 minutes.

Makes 20 cookies

NUTRIENT IQ POINTS: 13 per cookie

CALORIES 211; PROTEIN 6g; CARBOHYDRATES 28g; SUGARS 13g; TOTAL FAT 9.5g; SATURATED FAT 3.2g; CHOLESTEROL 0.3mg; SODIUM 5mg; FIBER 5.8g; BETA-CAROTENE 12ug; VITAMIN C 1mg; CALCIUM 45mg; IRON 3.8mg; FOLATE 49ug; MAGNESIUM 63mg; POTASSIUM 295mg; ZINC 1mg; SELENIUM 2.2ug

CHAPTER 1

1.   Health, United States 2019. Table 44. Gross domestic product, national health expenditures, per capita amounts, percent distribution, and average annual percent change: United States, selected years 1960–2018. 2019.

2.   Centers for Medicare & Medicaid Services. National Health Expenditure Data. [https://www.cms.gov Research Statistics-Data-and-Systems/StatisticsTrends and-Reports/NationalHealthExpendData NationalHealthAccountsHistorical]

3.   Ostbye T, Stroo M, Eisenstein EL, et al. Is overweight and class I obesity associated with increased health claims costs? *Obesity (Silver Spring)* 2014, **22**:1179-1186.

4.   Collaborators GBDD. Health effects of dietary risks in 195 countries, 1990-2017: a systematic analysis for the Global Burden of Disease Study 2017. *Lancet* 2019.

5.   Hales CM, Carroll MD, Fryar CD, Ogden CL. Prevalence of Obesity and Severe Obesity Among Adults: United States, 2017-2018. *NCHS Data Brief* 2020:1-8.

6.   Fryar CD, Carroll MD, Ogden CL. Prevalence of Overweight, Obesity, and Severe Obesity Among Adults Aged 20 and Over: United States, 1960–1962 Through 2015–2016. *NATIONAL CENTER FOR HEALTH STATISTICS Health E-Stats* 2018.

7. Ogden CL, Fryar CD, Carroll MD, Flegal KM. **Mean body weight, height, and body mass index, United States 1960-2002.** *Adv Data* 2004:1-17.

8. Fryar CD, Carroll MD, Gu Q, et al. **Anthropometric Reference Data for Children and Adults: United States, 2015 2018.** *Vital Health Stat 3* 2021:1-44.

9. **Per capita consumption of soft drinks in the United States from 2010 to 2018** [https://www.statista.com/statistics/306836/us-percapita-consumption-of-softdrinks/]

10. **Loss-adjusted food availability. Food Availability (Per Capita) Data System. U.S. Department of Agriculture, Economic Research Service.** 2021.

11. **U.S. Department of Agriculture, Agricultural Research Service. Energy Intakes: Percentages of Energy from Protein, Carbohydrate, Fat, and Alcohol, by Gender and Age, What We Eat in America, NHANES 2017-2018.** 2020.

12. **Food and Agriculture Organization of the United Nations. Food Balances.**

13. Kuck G, Schnitkey G: **An Overview of Meat Consumption in the United States.** In *Farmdoc daily*, vol. 11: Department of Agricultural and Consumer Economics, University of Illinois at Urbana-Champaign; 2021.

14. Gu Q, Paulose-Ram R, Burt VL, Kit BK. **Prescription cholesterol-lowering medication use in adults aged 40 and over: United States, 2003 2012.** *NCHS Data Brief* 2014:1-8.

15. Reider CA, Chung RY, Devarshi PP, et al. **Inadequacy of Immune Health Nutrients: Intakes in US Adults, the 2005-2016 NHANES.** *Nutrients* 2020, **12.**

16. Fulgoni VL, 3rd, Keast DR, Bailey RL, Dwyer J. **Foods, fortificants, and supplements: Where do Americans get their nutrients?** *J Nutr* 2011, **141**:1847 1854.

17. Wing RR, Phelan S. **Long-term weight loss maintenance.** *Am J Clin Nutr* 2005, **82**:222S-225S.

18. Ayyad C, Andersen T. **Long-term efficacy of dietary treatment of obesity: a systematic review of studies published between 1931 and 1999.** *Obes Rev* 2000, **1**:113 119.

19. Fuhrman J, Sarter B, Glaser D, Acocella S. **Changing perceptions of hunger on a high nutrient density diet.** *Nutr J* 2010, **9**:51.

20. Slavin JL. **Dietary fiber and body weight.** *Nutrition* 2005, **21**:411-418.

21. Davis JN, Hodges VA, Gillham MB. **Normal weight adults consume more fiber and fruit than their age- and height-matched overweight/obese counterparts.** *J Am Diet Assoc* 2006, **106**:833-840.

22. Huang RY, Huang CC, Hu FB, Chavarro JE. **Vegetarian Diets and Weight Reduction: a Meta Analysis of Randomized Controlled Trials.** *J Gen Intern Med* 2016, **31**:109-116.

23. Ello-Martin JA, Roe LS, Ledikwe JH, et al. **Dietary energy density in the treatment of obesity: a year-long trial comparing 2 weight-loss diets.** *Am J Clin Nutr* 2007, **85**:1465-1477.

24. Dreher ML, Ford NA. **A Comprehensive Critical Assessment of Increased Fruit and Vegetable Intake on Weight Loss in Women.** *Nutrients* 2020, **12**.

CHAPTER 3

1. Centers for Disease Control and Prevention. **Safer and healthier foods.** *MMWR Morb Mortal Wkly Rep* 1999, **48**:905-913.

2. Collaborators GBDD. **Health effects of dietary risks in 195 countries, 1990-2017: a systematic analysis for the Global Burden of Disease Study 2017.** *Lancet* 2019.

3. Heron M. **Deaths: Leading Causes for 2019.** *Natl Vital Stat Rep* 2021, **70**:1-114.

4. Liu RH. **Health-promoting components of fruits and vegetables in the diet.** *Adv Nutr* 2013, **4**:384S-392S.

5. Patra S, Nayak R, Patro S, et al. **Chemical diversity of dietary phytochemicals and their mode of chemoprevention.** *Biotechnol Rep (Amst)* 2021, 30:e00633.

6. Weiss JF, Landauer MR. **Protection against ionizing radiation by antioxidant nutrients and phytochemicals.** *Toxicology* 2003, **189**:1-20.

7. Ornish D, Brown SE, Scherwitz LW, et al. **Can lifestyle changes reverse coronary heart disease? The Lifestyle Heart Trial.** *Lancet* 1990, **336**:129 133.

8. Ornish D, Scherwitz LW, Billings JH, et al. **Intensive lifestyle changes for reversal of coronary heart disease.** *JAMA* 1998, **280**:2001-2007. Esselstyn CB, Jr., Ellis SG, Medendorp SV, Crowe TD. **A strategy to arrest and reverse coronary artery disease: a 5-year longitudinal study of a single physician's practice.** *J Fam Pract* 1995, **41**:560-568.

9. Casas R, Castro-Barquero S, Estruch R, Sacanella E. **Nutrition and Cardiovascular Health.** *Int J Mol Sci* 2018, **19**.

10. Fuhrman J, Singer M. **Improved Cardiovascular Parameter With a Nutrient-Dense, Plant-Rich Diet-Style: A Patient Survey With Illustrative Cases.** *Am J Lifestyle Med* 2017, **11**:264-273.

11. Chiavaroli L, Nishi SK, Khan TA, et al. **Portfolio=Dietary Pattern and Cardiovascular Disease: ASystematic Review and Meta-analysis of Controlled Trials.** *Prog Cardiovasc Dis* 2018, **61**:43-53.

12. Patel H, Chandra S, Alexander S, et al. **Plant-Based Nutrition: An Essential Component of Cardiovascular Disease Prevention and Management.** *Curr Cardiol Rep* 2017, **19**:104.

13. Most J, Tosti V, Redman LM, Fontana L. **Calorie restriction in humans: An update.** *Ageing Res Rev* 2017,39:36-45.

CHAPTER 4

1. **U.S. Centers for Disease Control and Prevention: Sodium and Food Sources** [https://www.cdc.gov/salt/food.htm]

FOR MORE INFORMATION, VISIT:

www.DrFuhrman.com

Dr. Fuhrman's official website for information, recipes, supportive services, and products

OR CALL:

800-474-WELL (9355)

Membership

DrFuhrman.com provides a roadmap for your wellness journey. You'll find the guidance, practical tips, recipes, meal plans, and educational resources you need to make the Nutritarian lifestyle easy and enjoyable.

Membership levels

Gold (monthly / annual)
Platinum (monthly / annual)
Diamond (lifetime)

Recipes and Meal Plans

Enjoy 2,000+ delicious recipes, meal plans and recipe collections. Each printable recipe includes ingredient lists, instructions, and tips for flavoring your dishes without salt. New recipes added regularly. Meal Plans are available to help you meet specific health goals.

Ask the Doctor

Communicate directly with Dr. Fuhrman by posting your health personal health questions in the ASK THE DOCTOR forum. (You will be able to create a screen name for privacy.) Dr. Fuhrman monitors the forum daily, and provides valuable insights. (Platinum, Diamond level required for posting; all members may search the archive.)

Product Discounts

Members receive a 10% discount on all Dr. Fuhrman brand supplements and up to a 25% discount on all Dr. Fuhrman foods and select books and media.

My Health Tracker

Use this online tool to record your health history and chart your progress as you follow the Nutritarian diet.

Position Papers and Media

In-depth analysis of topics such as IGF-1 and cancer; mammograms; folate; protein; Parkinson's Disease and more. Members may download papers for free, and view the library of videos and teleconferences.

Nutritarian Network Private Group

Connect with others who share your wellness goals in this members'-only forum.

For more details on the benefits of membership, visit www.drfuhrman.com/membership